www.harcourt-international.com

Bringing you products from all Harcourt Health Sciences companies including Baillière Tindall, Churchill Livingstone, Mosby and W.B. Saunders

- ▶ **Browse** for latest information on new books, journals and electronic products

- ▶ **Search** for information on over 20 000 published titles with full product information including tables of contents and sample chapters

- ▶ **Keep up to date** with our extensive publishing programme in your field by registering with **eAlert** or requesting postal updates

- ▶ **Secure online ordering** with prompt delivery, as well as full contact details to order by phone, fax or post

- ▶ **News** of special features and promotions

If you are based in the following countries, please visit the country-specific site to receive full details of product availability and local ordering information

USA: www.harcourthealth.com

Canada: www.harcourtcanada.com

Australia: www.harcourt.com.au

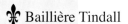 Baillière Tindall   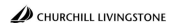 CHURCHILL LIVINGSTONE   Mosby   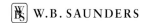 W.B. SAUNDERS

WW 160 KAN   43606 (1) 49.99

Systemic
Diseases
and the Eye

Commissioning Editor: *Sue Hodgson*
Project Development Manager: *Francesca Lumkin*
Project Manager: *Cheryl Brant*
Design Manager: *Jayne Jones*
Illustrations Manager: *Mick Ruddy*
Page Make-up: *Alan Palfreyman*

Systemic Diseases and the Eye

Signs and differential diagnosis

Jack J Kanski MD MS FRCS FRCOphth

Consultant Ophthalmic Surgeon
Prince Charles Eye Unit
King Edward VII Hospital
Windsor
UK

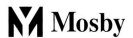 Mosby

London • Edinburgh • New York • Philadelphia • St Louis • Sydney • Toronto 2001

MOSBY
An imprint of Mosby International Limited

First published 2001

ISBN 0 7234 3216 3

British Library Cataloguing in Publication Data
A catalogue record for this book is available from the British Library

Library of Congress Cataloging in Publication Data
A catalog record for this book is available from the Library of Congress

Note
Medical knowledge is constantly changing. As new information becomes available,
changes in treatment, procedures, equipment and the use of drugs become necessary. The
editors/authors/contributors and the publishers have taken care to ensure that the information given in this text is accurate and up to date. However, readers are strongly advised to
confirm that the information, especially with regard to drug usage, complies with the latest legislation and standards of practice.

Existing UK nomenclature is changing to the system of Recommended International Non-
proprietary Names (rINNs). Until the UK names are no longer in use, these more familiar
names are used in this book in preference to rINNs, details of which may be obtained
from the British National Formulary.

Printed in China

The
Publisher's
policy is to use
**paper manufactured
from sustainable forests**

CONTENTS

Part One: Differential Diagnosis of Eye Signs

Part Two: Differential Diagnosis of Systemic Signs

Part Three: Systemic Features and Eyes Signs

Contents

PREFACE

It is surprising how many systemic diseases have potential ocular manifestations or associations. In some cases ocular manifestations are common and potentially serious, e.g. in diabetes, whilst in others they are uncommon and innocuous, e.g. in gout. The purpose of this book is twofold. The first is to remind practising ophthalmologists of the many diverse physical signs of systemic conditions that may affect the eye. The second is to acquaint the non-ophthalmologist with potential ocular manifestations of systemic diseases. Only those diseases that may be of interest to the general physician have been included, so that rare pediatric disorders and syndromes have not been described; systemic conditions without ocular associations have also not been included.

Systemic Diseases and the Eye is divided into three parts which should be read sequentially. The first part describes the various eye signs, starting with the eyelids and finishing with ophthalmoplegia. The potential systemic association of each sign is indicated together with its most important systemic clinical features. The second part describes the various systemic signs, starting with the face and finishing with the nervous system. The potential ocular associations of each systemic disease are indicated in order of importance. The third part summarizes both the systemic and ocular signs of each disease mentioned in the book. The important or common ocular manifestations are indicated in italic type. Icons have been used throughout the book for quicker reference.

Jack J. Kanski
2001

GUIDE TO ICONS

Signs

Complications

Presentation

Systemic Features

Eye signs

Causes

Look for

Associations

ACKNOWLEDGEMENTS

I would like to thank **Anne Bolton** for taking many of the photographs, and also to the following colleagues and photographic departments for supplying additional material, without which this book could not have been written:

C. Barry, Lions Eye Institute, Perth, W. Australia (Figures 1.139, 2.16)

K. Bibby (Figure 1.98)

A. Chopdar (Figure 3.256)

A. Cruess (Figure 1.132)

B. Damato (Figures 1.133, 3.117)

S. Dawson (Figure 2.97)

T. ffytche (Figures 2.145, 3.107)

Professor A. Fielder (Figure 1.67)

P. Frith (Figure 1.100)

S. Ford, Western Eye Hospital (Figures 1.75, 1.76, 1.87, 1.89, 1.101, 1.105, 1.134, 1.141, 2.130, 3.9, 3.11, 3.116, 3.136, 3.144, 3.149, 3.202)

S. Giacy (Figure 3.226)

J. Govan (Figures 1.66, 3.12)

Professor B. Jay (Figure 1.123)

Professor S. Lightman (Figure 1.108)

S. Milewski (Figure 1.131)

S. Mitchell (Figures 1.111, 3.5)

Moorfields Eye Hospital (Figure 3.88)

P. Morse (Figures 1.83, 3.55, 3.122, 3.203, 3.220)

K. Nischal (Figures 2.147, 2.150, 3.76, 3.143, 3.152, 3.184, 3.185, 3.242, 3.243, 3.252)

B. Noble (Figures 1.106, 2.192, 3.25, 3.26, 3.30)

T. Rahman (Figure 1.114)

G. Rose (Figures 3.30, 3.33)

Royal Free Hospital (Figure 3.50)

Royal Victoria Infirmary, Newcastle, (Figure 1.126)

J. Salmon (Figures 2.148, 3.220)

Southampton General Hospital, Eye Department (Figure 1.45)

D. Thomas (Figure 3.1).

1 Differential Diagnosis of Eye Signs

THE EYELIDS

Ptosis

Signs

- Ptosis is a drooping of the upper eyelid so that the lower lid margin is located more than two millimeters below the limbus.

Systemic Associations

1. Third nerve palsy

 Signs

- Ptosis is unilateral and usually moderate to severe (**Fig. 1.1**).
- In the primary position the eye is slightly divergent and depressed.
- Limitation of adduction, elevation and depression.
- Paralysis of accommodation.
- The pupil may or may not be fixed and dilated depending on the cause.

 Look for

- *If the pupil is uninvolved* – diabetes and hypertension.
- *If the pupil is involved* – posterior communicating aneurysm.

2. Horner syndrome

 Signs

- Mild unilateral ptosis (**Fig. 1.2**).
- Ipsilateral miosis.
- Ipsilateral slight elevation of the lower eyelid.

- Ipsilateral reduction in sweating if the lesion is below the superior cervical ganglion.
- Heterochromia iridis may be present if the lesion is congenital, or acquired and longstanding.

 Look for

- *In central lesions* – brainstem disease and syringomyelia.
- *In preganglionic lesions* – Pancoast tumor, aortic artery disease and neck lesions.
- *In postganglionic lesions* – cluster headache, nasopharyngeal tumor and internal carotid artery disease.

3. Myasthenia gravis

 Signs

- Ptosis is usually insidious, bilateral but frequently asymmetrical. It is worse with fatigue and in upgaze (**Fig. 1.3**).

 Look for

- Intermittent vertical diplopia.
- Excessive muscular fatiguability, particularly involving the arms and proximal muscles of the legs.
- Problems with speech, chewing and swallowing.

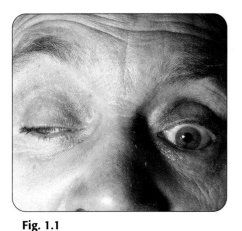

Fig. 1.1

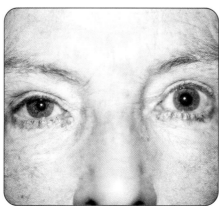

Fig. 1.2

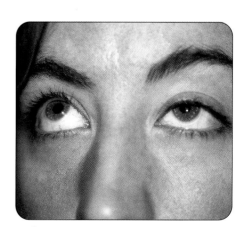

Fig. 1.3

4. Myotonic dystrophy

 Signs

- Ptosis is bilateral and mild to moderate (**Fig. 1.4**).

 Look for

- Mournful facial expression.
- Myotonia of peripheral muscles making release of grip difficult.
- Hypogonadism resulting in infertility or sterility.

5. Ocular myopathies

 Signs

- Ptosis is symmetrical and progressive (**Fig. 1.5**).
- Progressive symmetrical external ophthalmoplegia.

 Look for

- *Primary ocular myopathy*.
- *Oculopharyngeal dystrophy* – weakness of pharyngeal muscles and wasting of the temporalis.

- *Kearns–Sayre syndrome* – pigmentary retinopathy, heart block and ataxia.

6. Bassen–Kornzweig syndrome

 Signs

- Ptosis is symmetrical and progressive.

 Look for

- Pigmentary retinopathy.
- Steatorrhea and malabsorption.
- Spinocerebellar ataxia.

7. Eaton–Lambert myasthenic syndrome

 Signs

- Bilateral ptosis.

 Look for

- Diplopia.
- Limb weakness and abnormal gait.
- Small-cell bronchial carcinoma.

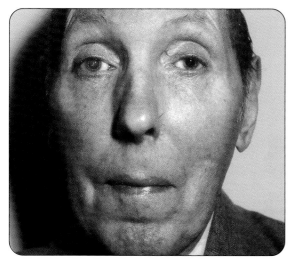

Fig. 1.4

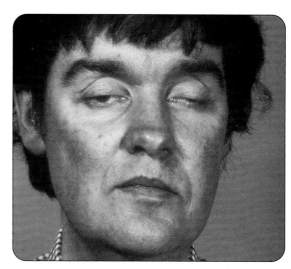

Fig. 1.5

Lid Retraction

Definition

- In lid retraction the lower margin of the upper eyelid is either level with or above the limbus.

Systemic Associations

1. Thyrotoxicosis

 Signs

- Lid retraction is usually bilateral but may be asymmetrical (**Fig. 1.6**).

 Look for

- Thyroid enlargement.
- Fine tremor of the hands.
- Tachycardia and atrial fibrillation.

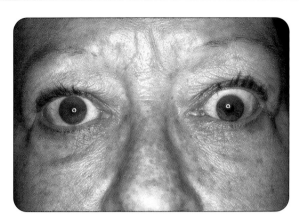

Fig. 1.6

2. Parinaud dorsal midbrain syndrome

 Signs

- Lid retraction is usually symmetrical (**Fig. 1.7**).
- Supranuclear upgaze palsy.
- Large pupils with light–near dissociation.
- Paralysis of convergence.
- Convergence–retraction nystagmus.

 Look for

- *In children* – aqueduct stenosis, meningitis and pinealoma.
- *In young adults* – demyelination, trauma and arteriovenous fistula.
- *In the elderly* – midbrain vascular accidents, tumor and aneurysm.

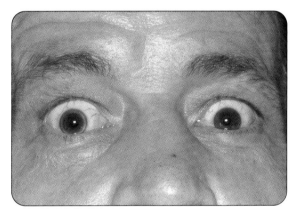

Fig. 1.7

Xanthelasma

Signs

- Bilateral, yellowish subcutaneous plaques usually located medially (**Fig. 1.8**).

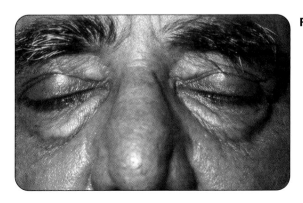

Fig. 1.8

Systemic Associations

1. Primary hyperlipoproteinemia

 Look for

- Tendon xanthomata.
- Atherosclerosis.

2. Primary biliary cirrhosis

 Look for

- Secondary hypercholesterolemia.

- Jaundice and hepatosplenomegaly.
- Spider nevi and palmar erythema.

3. Cerebrotendinous xanthomatosis

 Look for

- Premature atherosclerosis.
- Tendon xanthomata and mental deterioration.
- Cerebellar ataxia and pyramidal signs.

THE ORBIT

Proptosis

Signs

- Proptosis is a forward displacement of the globe (**Fig. 1.9**). It may be unilateral or bilateral, and axial or non-axial.

- Congestive proptosis is characterized by associated pain, lid edema, chemosis, conjunctival congestion and ocular motility restriction (**Fig. 1.10**).

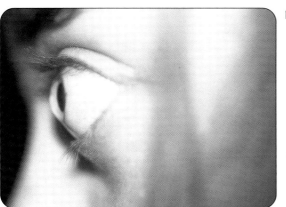

Fig. 1.9

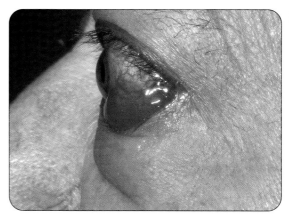

Fig. 1.10

Systemic Associations

1. Thyrotoxicosis

 Signs

- Congestive or non-congestive proptosis which may be unilateral or bilateral (**Fig. 1.11**).

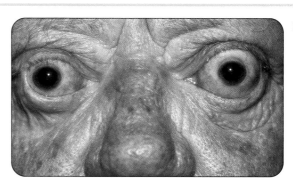

Fig. 1.11

Look for

- Thyroid enlargement.
- Fine tremor of the hands.
- Tachycardia and atrial fibrillation.

2. Carotid-cavernous fistula

 Signs

- Acute, unilateral, congestive, pulsatile proptosis associated with a bruit (**Fig. 1.12**).

 Look for

- Head trauma causing a basal skull fracture.
- Spontaneous rupture of an intracavernous aneurysm.

3. Wegener granulomatosis (Fig. 1.13).

 Signs

- Chonic, unilateral or bilateral, congestive proptosis.

 Look for

- Sinus inflammation and saddle-shaped nose.

- Lung cavitation.
- Necrotizing glomerulonephritis.

4. Non-Hodgkin lymphoma

 Signs

- Chronic, unilateral or bilateral proptosis (**Fig. 1.14**).

 Look for

- Weight loss and fever.
- Asymptomatic lymphadenopathy.

5. Metastatic carcinoma

 Signs

- Acute, unilateral proptosis and ophthalmoplegia (**Fig. 1.15**).

 Look for

- Primary sites – breast, bronchus, prostate, skin melanoma, gastrointestinal tract and kidney.

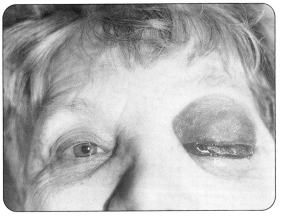

Fig. 1.12

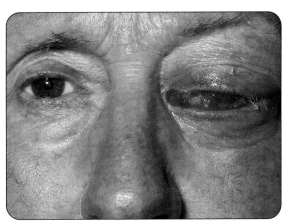

Fig. 1.13

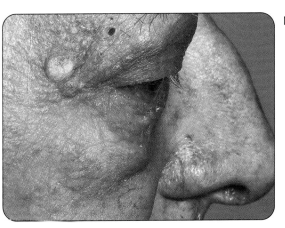

Fig. 1.14

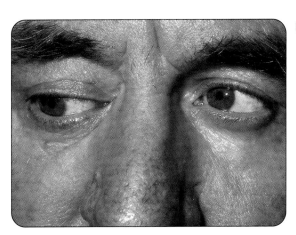

Fig. 1.15

6. Neurofibromatosis-1 (optic nerve glioma)

 Signs

- Chronic, unilateral, non-congestive proptosis (**Fig. 1.16**).

 Look for

- *Neural tumors* – brain and peripheral nerves.
- *Skin lesions* – café-au-lait spots, freckles, fibroma molluscum and plexiform neurofibromas.
- *Skeletal defects* – scoliosis, absence of the greater wing of the sphenoid bone and facial hemiatrophy.

7. Acute leukemia in children

 Signs

- Unilateral or bilateral, congestive or non-congestive proptosis (**Fig. 1.17**).

 Look for

- Purpura and easy bruising.
- Lymphadenopathy and splenomegaly.

8. Hand–Schüller–Christian disease

 Signs

- Unilateral or bilateral non-congestive proptosis.

 Look for

- Diabetes insipidus and lytic bone lesions.
- Pulmonary disease with hilar adenopathy.

9. Other
- Polyarteritis nodosa.
- Multiple myeloma.
- Waldenström macroglobulinemia.
- Paget disease.
- Cushing syndrome.

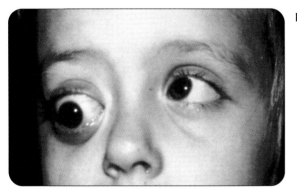

Fig. 1.16

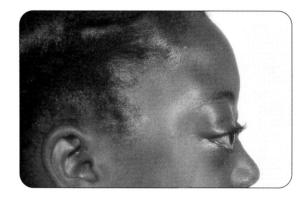

Fig. 1.17

THE LACRIMAL GLAND

Keratoconjunctivitis sicca

Signs

- Corneal filaments (**Fig. 1.18**).

- Staining of the conjunctiva and corneal filaments with rose bengal (**Fig. 1.19**).

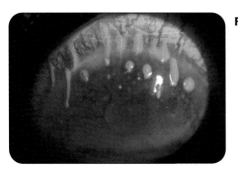

Fig. 1.18

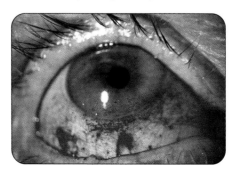

Fig. 1.19

Systemic Associations

1. Primary Sjögren syndrome

 Look for

- Xerostomia, dry nasal passages and diminished vaginal secretions.
- Cutaneous vasculitis.
- Raynaud phenomenon.

2. Rheumatoid arthritis

 Look for

- Symmetrical, erosive polyarthritis.
- Subcutaneous nodules.
- Cutaneous vascultitis.

3. Systemic lupus erythematosus

 Look for

- Facial rash with a characteristic 'butterfly' distribution.
- Cutaneous vasculitis and photosensitivity.
- Glomerulonephritis.

4. Primary biliary cirrhosis

 Look for

- Secondary hypercholesterolemia.
- Jaundice and hepatosplenomegaly.
- Spider nevi and palmar erythema.

5. Systemic sclerosis

 Look for

- Raynaud phenomenon.
- Waxy and tight skin appearance (acrosclerosis).
- Esophageal dysmobility.

6. Dermatomyositis and polymyositis

 Look for

- Widespread erythematous skin rash.
- Weakness and atrophy of proximal limb muscles.
- Subcutaneous calcification with ulceration.

7. Relapsing polychondritis

 Look for

- Destruction of the pinnae and saddle-shaped nose.
- Stridor due to involvement of the larynx and trachea.
- Polyarthritis.

8. Other
- AIDS.
- Hemochromatosis.
- Mixed connective tissue disease.
- Longstanding thyroid disease.
- Familial dysautonomia (Riley–Day syndrome).

THE CONJUNCTIVA

Conjunctivitis

Signs

- Conjunctival hyperemia which is least at the limbus and maximal in the fornices.
- The conjunctival reaction may be follicular, papillary or non-specific, depending on the cause.
- The discharge may be watery, mucoid, purulent or mucopurulent.
- Conjunctival membrane or pseudomembrane formation may occur in certain cases.

Systemic Associations

1. Reiter syndrome

 Signs

- Bilateral, acute, mucopurulent conjunctivitis (**Fig. 1.20**).

 Look for

- Urethritis.
- Asymmetrical arthritis most frequently involving the knees and ankles.
- Circinate balanitis.
- Keratoderma blennorrhagica involving the palms and soles.

2. Atopic eczema

 Signs

- Bilateral, chronic, papillary conjunctivitis (**Fig. 1.21**).

 Look for

- Dry, erythematous thickening of the skin of the face, side of the neck, and flexure surfaces of the wrists, ankles, elbows and knees.

3. Chlamydial genital infection

 Signs

- Unilateral or bilateral, subacute follicular conjunctivitis and regional lymphadenopathy (**Fig. 1.22**).

 Look for

a. *In males* – 'non-specific urethritis'.
b. *In females* – abacterial pyuria and cervicitis.

4. Thyrotoxicosis

 Signs

- Usually bilateral but asymmetrical, chronic, papillary, superior limbic keratoconjunctivitis (**Fig. 1.23**).

 Look for

- Thyroid enlargement.
- Fine tremor of the hands.
- Tachycardia and atrial fibrillation.

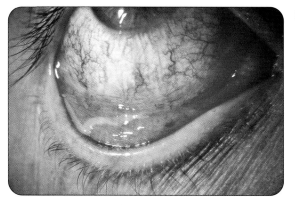

Fig. 1.20

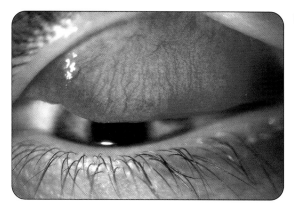

Fig. 1.21

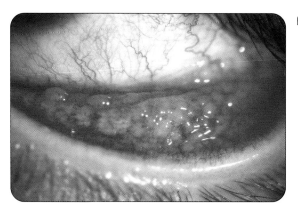

Fig. 1.22

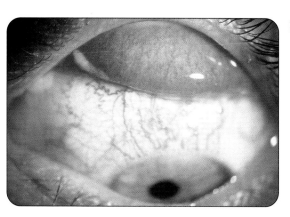

Fig. 1.23

5. Early Stevens–Johnson syndrome

 Signs

- Bilateral, subacute, membraneous conjunctivitis (**Fig. 1.24**).

 Look for

- Oral bullae with hemorrhagic crusting of the lips.
- Cutaneous bullae.
- Target skin lesions involving the palms and soles.

6. Gonorrhea

 Signs

- Bilateral, hyperacute, purulent conjunctivitis with edema of the eyelids and regional lymphadenopathy (**Fig. 1.25**).

 Look for

- *In males* – urethral discharge and dysuria.

- *In females* – vaginal discharge and less frequently dysuria.

7. Kawasaki syndrome

 Signs

- Bilateral acute conjunctivitis.

 Look for

- Erythematous rash.
- Pancarditis, coronary disease and aneurysm formation.
- Indurative edema of the extremities.

8. Other
- Lyme disease stage 1.
- Ulcerative colitis.
- Crohn disease.
- Pemphigus vulgaris.

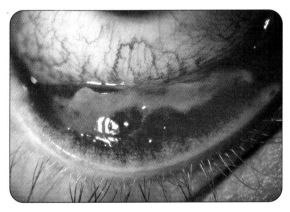

Fig. 1.24

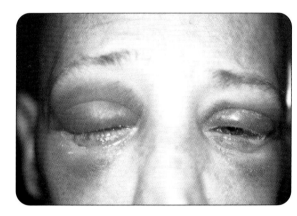

Fig. 1.25

Conjunctival cicatrization

Signs

- Symblepharon (**Fig. 1.26**).
- Eventual obliteration of the fornices (**Fig. 1.27**).
- Keratopathy (**Fig. 1.28**).

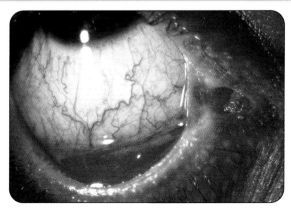

Fig. 1.26

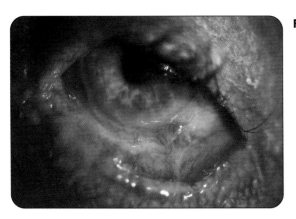

Fig. 1.27

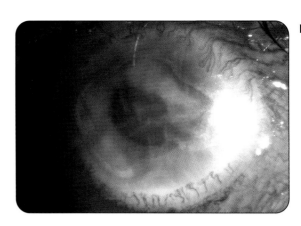

Fig. 1.28

Systemic Associations

1. Cicatricial pemphigoid

 Look for

- Mucosal blisters which most frequently involve the mouth.
- Skin blisters which are usually sparse and heal by scarring.

2. Late Stevens–Johnson syndrome

 Look for

- The mucocutaneous lesions have usually resolved when conjunctival cicatrization develops.

3. Epidermolysis bullosa

 Look for

- Skin blistering which is induced by trauma.
- Mitten-hands and feet with partial syndactyly.

4. Porphyria cutanea tarda

 Look for

- Skin blistering which follows exposure to sunlight.
- Skin hyperpigmentation.

5. Toxic epidermal necrolysis (Lyell disease, scalded skin syndrome)

 Look for

- Mucosal blistering which is universal.
- Transient, widespread, painful skin blistering which resembles scalded skin.

6. Linear IgA disease (bullous dermatosis)

 Look for

- Tense mucocutaneous blisters.

7. Pemphigoid

 Look for

- Mucosal blisters which are frequent.
- Large, symmetrical, widespread but self-limiting skin blisters.

8. Dermatitis herpetiformis

 Look for

- Groups of small skin blisters associated with urticaria.

Parinaud oculoglandular syndrome

Signs

- Conjunctival granulomas and large follicles (**Fig. 1.29**).
- Severe preauricular or submandibular lymphadenopathy.

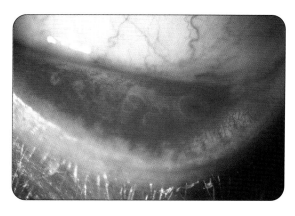

Fig. 1.29

Systemic Associations

1. Cat-scratch fever

 Look for

- Fever and malaise.
- Skin papule and regional lymphadenopathy.

2. Lymphogranuloma venereum

 Look for

- Painless genital ulceration.
- Painful regional lymphadenopathy.

3. Chancroid

 Look for

- Painful genital ulceration.
- Regional lymphadenopathy which may become suppurated.

Conjunctival vascular abnormalities

Systemic Associations

1. Carotid-cavernous fistula

 Signs

- Severe, generalized, epibulbar vascular dilatation and tortuosity (**Fig. 1.30**).
- Associated congestive, pulsatile proptosis associated with a bruit.

 Look for

- Head trauma causing a basal skull fracture.
- Spontaneous fracture of an intracavernous aneurysm.

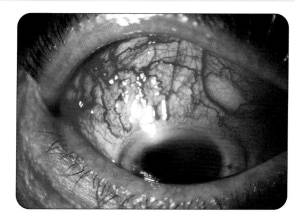

Fig. 1.30

2. Sturge–Weber syndrome

 Signs

- Episcleral hemangioma (**Fig. 1.31**).
- Associated ipsilateral nevus flammeus.

 Look for

- Ipsilateral leptomeningeal hemangioma.
- Contralateral hemiparesis or hemianopia.
- Epilepsy.

3. Ataxia telangiectasia (Louis–Bar syndrome)

 Signs

- Bulbar conjunctival telangiectasia (**Fig. 1.32**).

 Look for

- Skin telangiectasia involving the pinnae, face and limb flexures.
- Ataxia and choreoathetosis.

4. Rendu–Osler–Weber disease (hereditary hemorrhagic telangiectasia)

 Signs

- Conjunctival telangiectasia.

 Look for

- Telangiectasia of the skin, lips and tongue.
- Arteriovenous malformations in the lungs and gastrointestinal system which may bleed.

5. Fabry disease

 Signs

- Conjunctival telangiectasia.

 Look for

- Purple telangiectatic skin lesions (angiokeratomas).
- Cardiovascular, renal and pulmonary disease.

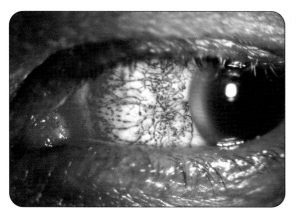

Fig. 1.31

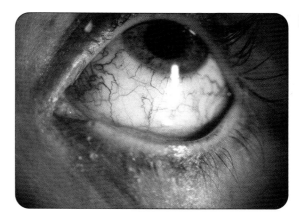

Fig. 1.32

THE SCLERA

Anterior scleritis

Signs

- *Non-necrotizing scleritis* is characterized by congestion of the deep vascular plexus and may be nodular (**Fig. 1.33**) or diffuse (**Fig. 1.34**).
- *Necrotizing with inflammation* is characterized by avascular patches (**Fig. 1.35**).

- *Scleromalacia perforans* is characterized by gross scleral thinning with exposure of underlying uveal tissue (**Fig. 1.36**). It occurs exclusively in patients with rheumatoid arthritis.

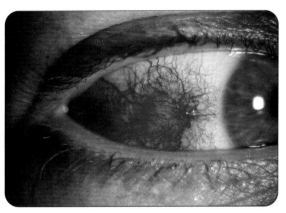

Fig. 1.33

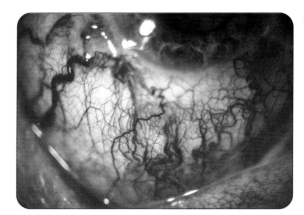

Fig. 1.34

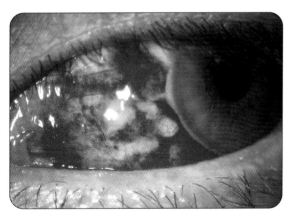

Fig. 1.35

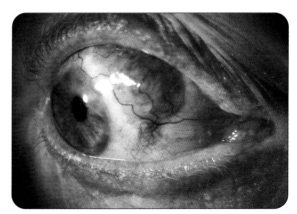

Fig. 1.36

Systemic Associations

1. Rheumatoid arthritis

 Look for

- Symmetrical erosive polyarthritis.
- Subcutaneous nodules.
- Cutaneous vasculitis.

2. Wegener granulomatosis

 Look for

- Sinus inflammation and saddle-shaped nose.
- Lung cavitation.
- Necrotizing glomerulonephritis.

3. Systemic lupus erythematosus

 Look for

- Facial rash with a characteristic 'butterfly' distribution.
- Cutaneous vasculitis and photosensitivity.
- Glomerulonephritis.

4. Polyarteritis nodosa

 Look for

- Arthralgia and myalgia.
- Purpura, easy bruising and cutaneous vasculitis.
- Renal and cardiovascular disease.

5. Relapsing polychondritis

 Look for

- Destruction of the pinnae and saddle-shaped nose.
- Stridor due to involvement of the larynx and trachea.
- Polyarthritis.

6. Dermatomyositis – polymyositis

 Look for

- Widespread erythematous skin rash (only in dermato-myositis).
- Weakness and atrophy of proximal limb muscles.
- Subcutaneous calcification with ulceration.

7. Churg–Strauss syndrome

 Look for

- Pulmonary disease.
- Cutaneous vasculitis and subcutaneous nodules.
- Multifocal neuropathy.

8. Porphyria cutanea tarda

 Look for

- Bullous skin eruptions on exposure to sunlight.
- Skin hyperpigmentation.
- Hirsutism in females.

Blue sclera

Signs

- Blue sclera is caused by thinning and transparency of scleral collagen fibres that allow visualization of the underlying uvea (**Fig. 1.37**).

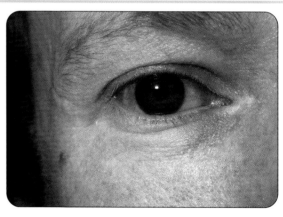

Fig. 1.37

Systemic Associations

1. Osteogenesis imperfecta types 1, 2 and 3

 Look for

- *Type 1* – joint hypermobility and cardiac valve lesions.
- *Type 2* – multiple fractures and short limbs.
- *Type 3* – bone deformity, dental hypoplasia and a trian-gular-shaped face.

2. Ehlers–Danlos syndrome type 6

 Look for

- Thin and hyperelastic skin which bruises easily and heals slowly.
- Joint hyperextensibility and easy dislocation.
- Dissecting aortic aneurysm and mitral valve disease.

Kayser–Fleischer ring

Signs

- Bilateral, circumferential, greenish-brown, peripheral band 1–3 mm in width located at the level of Descemet membrane (**Fig. 1.41**).

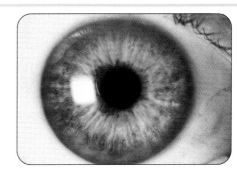

Fig. 1.41

Systemic association

1. Wilson disease

 Look for

- Liver disease and hepatosplenomegaly.

- Akinesis-rigidity syndrome with dyskinesis in childhood.
- Mental deterioration.

Corneal arcus

Signs

- Bilateral, circumferential, white, peripheral band about 1–2 mm in diameter with a diffuse central boundary located in the superficial corneal stroma (**Fig. 1.42**).

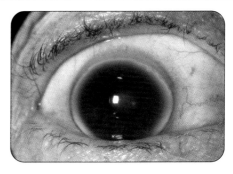

Fig. 1.42

Systemic Associations

1. Hyperlipoproteinemia

 Look for

- Tendon xanthomata.
- Atherosclerosis and coronary artery disease.

2. Lecithin–cholesterol–acetyltransferase deficiency

 Look for

- Early-onset atherosclerosis.
- Renal disease.
- Anemia.

3. Osteogenesis imperfecta type 1
(*see* Megalocornea p.18)

Corneal crystals

Signs

- Innumerable, minute glistening deposits within the epithelium, stroma, or both (**Fig. 1.43**).

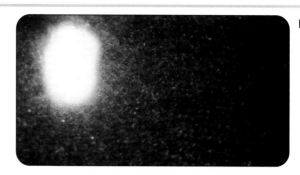

Fig. 1.43

Systemic Associations

1. Cystinosis

 Look for

- *Infantile nephropathic* – progressive nephropathy.
- *Non-nephropathic (adult)* – no nephropathy.
- *Intermediate (adolescent)* – variable nephropathy.

2. Multiple myeloma

 Look for

- Osteolytic bony lesions.
- Backache and pathologic fractures.
- Renal disease.

3. Waldenström macroglobulinemia

 Look for

- Lymphadenopathy and hepatosplenomegaly.
- Purpura.
- Peripheral vascular disease.

4. Tangier disease

 Look for

- Enlarged, orange colored tonsils and adenoids.
- Lemphadenopathy and hepatosplenomegaly.
- Thrombocytopenia.

5. Chronic gout
(*see* Band keratopathy p. 19)

Vortex keratopathy

Signs

- Bilateral, grayish or golden corneal epithelial deposits which appear in a vortex fashion from a point below the pupil and swirl outwards sparing the limbus (**Fig. 1.44**).

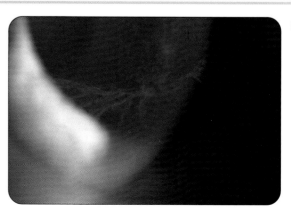

Fig. 1.44

Systemic Associations

1. Drug induced
- Amiodarone.
- Hydroxychloroquine and chloroquine.
- Indomethacin.
- Tamoxifen.
- Chlorpromazine.
- Mepacrine.
- Atovaquone.

2. Fabry disease

 Look for

- Purple telangiectatic skin lesions (angiokeratomas).
- Cardiovascular, renal and pulmonary disease.

Prominent corneal nerves

Signs

- Linear branching lines within the corneal stroma (**Fig. 1.45**).

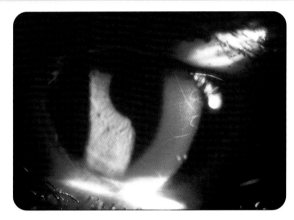

Fig. 1.45

Systemic Associations

1. Primary amyloidosis

 Look for

- Initially sensory and later motor peripheral neuropathy.
- Disease of the heart, kidneys, thyroid and adrenals.

2. Multiple endocrine neoplasia type IIb

 Look for

- Thickened lips and tongue.
- Marfanoid habitus.
- Thyroid carcinoma and pheochromocytoma.

3. Neurofibromatosis-1

 Look for

- *Neural tumors* – skin, brain, optic nerve, orbit, spine and autonomic nerves.
- *Skeletal defects* – scoliosis, congenital absence of the greater wing of the sphenoid bone, short stature and facial hemiatrophy.
- *Skin lesions* – café-au-lait spots, freckles and fibroma molluscum.

4. Refsum disease

 Look for

- Mixed motor and sensory polyneuropathy.
- Cerebellar ataxia, deafness and anosmia.
- Ichthyosis.

Peripheral ulcerative keratitis

Signs

- Corneal ulceration which progresses circumferentially and centrally (**Fig. 1.46**). In some cases the adjacent sclera may also be involved.

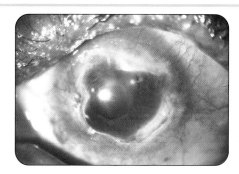

Fig. 1.46

Systemic Associations

1. Rheumatoid arthritis

 Look for

- Symmetrical, erosive polyarthritis.
- Subcutaneous nodules.
- Cutaneous vasculitis.

2. Wegener granulomatosis

 Look for

- Sinus inflammation and saddle-shaped nose.
- Lung cavitation.
- Necrotizing glomerulonephritis.

3. Polyarteritis nodosa

 Look for

- Arthralgia and myalgia.

- Purpura, easy bruising and cutaneous vasculitis.
- Renal and cardiovascular disease.

4. Systemic lupus erythematosus

 Look for

- Facial rash with a characteristic 'butterfly' distribution.
- Cutaneous vasculitis and photosensitivity.
- Glomerulonephritis.

5. Relapsing polychondritis

 Look for

- Destruction of the pinnae and saddle-shaped nose.
- Stridor due to involvement of the larynx and trachea.
- Polyarthritis.

Interstitial keratitis

Signs

- Midstromal, scarring and non-perfused 'ghost' vessels (**Fig. 1.47**).

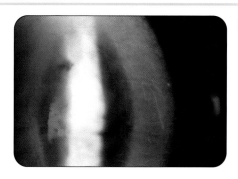

Fig. 1.47

Systemic Associations

1. Congential syphilis

 Look for

- Sensorineural deafness.
- Bone changes and saddle-shaped nose.
- Dental anomalies including malformed incisors (Hutchinson teeth) and mulberry molars.

2. Acquired syphilis

 Look for

- Maculopapular rash involving the trunk, palms and soles.
- Fever, malaise and generalized lymphadenopathy.

3. Lyme disease stage 3

 Look for

- Arthritis.
- Demyelinating encephalopathy.

4. Lymphogranuloma venereum

 Look for

- Painless genital ulceration.
- Painful regional lymphadenopathy.

5. Cogan syndrome

 Look for

- Acute-onset tinnitus, vertigo and deafness.

Inflammatory infiltrates

Systemic Associations

1. Chlamydial genital infection

 Signs

- Peripheral, subepithelial opacities associated with follicular conjunctivitis (**Fig. 1.48**).

 Look for

- *In males* – 'non-specific' urethritis.
- *In females* – abacterial pyuria and cervicitis.

2. Rosacea

 Signs

- Peripheral infiltrates, vascularization and thinning (**Fig. 1.49**).

 Look for

- Erythema and telangiectasia involving the glabella, cheeks, nose, and chin.

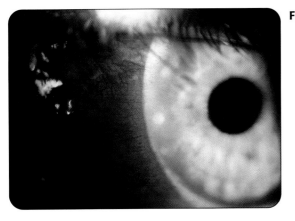

Fig. 1.48

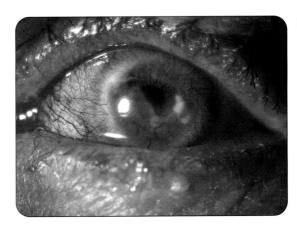

Fig. 1.49

3. Reiter syndrome

 Signs

- Subepithelial opacities in isolation or associated with conjunctivitis (**Fig. 1.50**).

 Look for

- Urethritis.
- Asymmetrical arthritis most frequently involving the knees and ankles.
- Circinate balanitis
- Keratoderma blennorrhagica involving the palms and soles.

4. Other

- AIDS (microsporidial keratitis).
- Crohn disease.
- Ulcerative colitis.

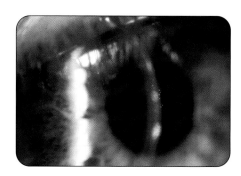

Fig. 1.50

THE IRIS

Non-granulomatous anterior uveitis

Signs

1. Acute anterior uveitis

- Circumcorneal injection and small pupil (**Fig. 1.51**).
- Small keratic precipitates on the endothelium ('dusting') (**Fig. 1.52**).
- Aqueous flare and cells (**Fig. 1.53**).
- Fibrinous exudate in the aqueous if severe (**Fig. 1.54**).
- Hypopyon if very severe (**Fig. 1.55**).

2. Chronic anterior uveitis

- Mild or absent circumcorneal injection.
- Small to medium-size keratic precipitates (**Fig. 1.56**).
- Aqueous flare and cells.
- Frequent posterior synechiae (**Fig. 1.57**).

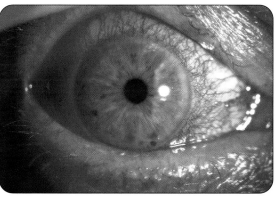

Fig. 1.51

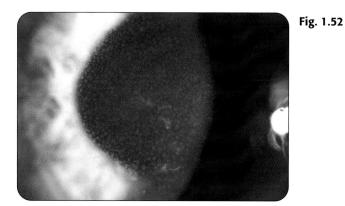

Fig. 1.52

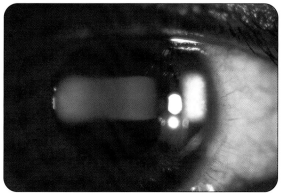

Fig. 1.53

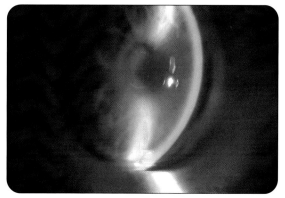

Fig. 1.54

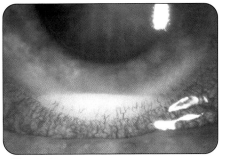

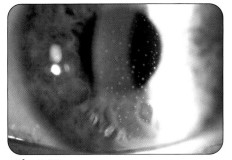

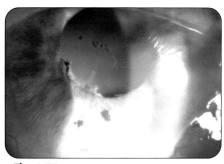

Fig. 1.55   Fig. 1.56   Fig. 1.57

Systemic Associations

1. Ankylosing spondylitis
- Acute anterior uveitis, frequently with a fibrinous exudate.

 Look for

- Pain and stiffness in the lower back or buttocks, more marked in the mornings.
- Limitation of spinal movements.

2. Reiter syndrome
- Acute, unilateral anterior uveitis.

 Look for

- Urethritis.
- Asymmetrical arthritis most frequently involving the knees and ankles.
- Circinate balanitis.
- Keratoderma blennorrhagica involving the palms and soles.

3. Behçet disease
- Acute anterior uveitis, frequently with a hypopyon.

 Look for

- Recurrent painful oral ulceration and genital ulceration.
- Cutaneous hypersensitivity, erythema nodosum and acneiform lesions.
- Recurrent thrombophlebitis.

4. Psoriatic arthritis
- Acute anterior uveitis.

 Look for

- Well-demarcated, scaly patches on extensor surfaces.
- Asymmetrical arthritis involving the knuckles and distal interphalangeal joints.
- Nail dystrophy.

5. Acute sarcoidosis
- Acute anterior uveitis.

 Look for

- *Löfgren syndrome* – fever, erythema nodosum and hilar lymphadenopathy.
- *Heerfordt syndrome* – fever and parotid enlargement.

6. Juvenile idiopathic arthritis
- Chronic anterior uveitis which is frequently bilateral.

 Look for

- Child under the age of 16 years.
- Arthritis is usually initially confined to five or fewer joints, most frequently the knees.

7. Ulcerative colitis
- Acute anterior uveitis.

 Look for

- Weight loss, fever and bloody diarrhea.
- Pyoderma gangrenosum and erythema nodosum.
- Liver disease and sclerosing cholangitis.

8. Crohn disease
- Acute anterior uveitis.

Look for

- Weight loss, diarrhea and abdominal pain.
- Perirectal fistulae and abscesses.
- Erythema nodosum and pyoderma gangrenosum.

9. Other
- Acquired syphilis.
- Kawasaki disease.
- Tubulointerstitial nephritis.
- IgA nephropathy.
- Leprosy.
- AIDS.
- Candidiasis.
- Coccidioidomycosis.
- Onchocerciasis.

Granulomatous anterior uveitis

Signs

- Mild or absent circumcorneal injection.
- Aqueous flare and cells.
- Large mutton-fat keratic precipitates (**Fig. 1.58**).
- Iris nodules (**Fig. 1.59**).
- Frequent posterior synechiae.

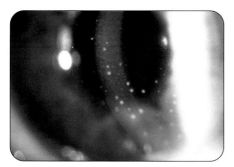

Fig. 1.58

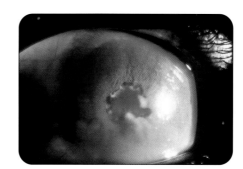

Fig. 1.59

Systemic Associations

1. Chronic sarcoidosis

 Look for

- *Cutaneous lesions* – lupus pernio and granulomas.
- *Pulmonary disease* – parenchymal infiltrates and fibrosis.
- *Neurological lesions* – multifocal peripheral neuropathy with a predilection for the facial nerve, meningeal infiltration and CNS granulomas.

2. Vogt–Koyanagi syndrome

 Look for

- Alopecia, poliosis and vitiligo.

3. Toxoplasmosis

- Also unifocal retinitis adjacent to an old scar.

 Look for

- *Congenital infestation (most common)* – no systemic features in adulthood.
- *Acquired infestation (rare)* – fever and lymphadenopathy.

4. Other

- Tuberculosis.
- Acquired syphilis.
- Leprosy.
- Non-Hodgkin large B-cell lymphoma.

Small non-inflammatory multifocal iris lesions

1. Brushfield spots

 Signs

- White or yellow spots arranged in a ring at the junction between the outer and middle third of the iris (**Fig. 1.60**).

 Look for

- Down syndrome.

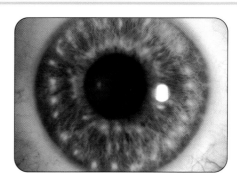

Fig. 1.60

2. Mammillations

 Signs

- Regularly spaced, tiny, smooth, villiform lesions (**Fig. 1.61**).

 Look for

- Nevus of Ota.
- Neurofibriomatosis-1.
- Rieger syndrome.

3. Lisch nodules

 Signs

- Small, brown, dome-shaped nodules (**Fig. 1.62**).

 Look for

- Neurofibromatosis-1.

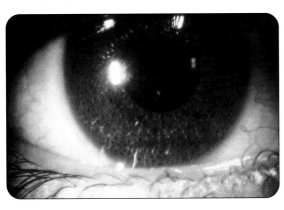

Fig. 1.61

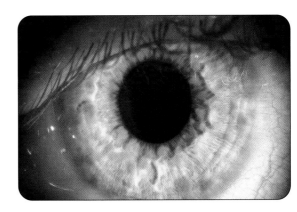

Fig. 1.62

Rubeosis iridis

Signs

- New blood vessels on the surface of the iris (**Fig. 1.63**).

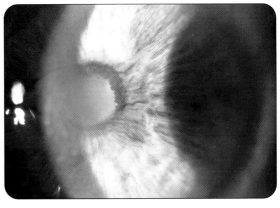

Fig. 1.63

Systemic Associations

1. Diabetes mellitus

 Look for

- Sensory polyneuropathy involving the feet.
- Accelerated atherosclerosis.
- Skin infections and necrobiosis lipoidica.

2. Ocular ischemic syndrome

 Look for

- Severe carotid stenosis.
- Direct carotid-cavernous fistula.
- Dissecting aortic aneurysm.
- Giant cells arteritis.
- Takayasu disease.

THE LENS

Lens displacement (ectopia lentis)

Signs

- Displacement of the lens from its normal position which may be partial (subluxation) or complete (dislocation or luxation).

Systemic Associations

1. Marfan syndrome
- Upward subluxation with preservation of the zonules (**Fig. 1.64**).

 Look for

- Tall and thin stature with disproportionally long limbs.
- Arachnodactyly and a high-arched palate.
- Aortic dilatation and mitral valve disease.

2. Homocystinuria
- Downward subluxation with disintegration of the zonules (**Fig. 1.65**).

 Look for

- Blond hair with a malar flush.
- Marfanoid habitus.
- Tendency to thromboses.

3. Weill–Marchesani syndrome

 Look for

- Short stature with small, stubby fingers (brachydactyly).
- Mental retardation.

4. Ehlers–Danlos syndrome type 6

 Look for

- Hyperelastic skin which bruises easily and heals slowly.
- Joint hyperextensibility and easy dislocation.
- Dissecting aneurysm and mitral valve disease.

5. Hyperlysinemia

 Look for

- Mental retardation.
- Lax ligaments and muscular hypotonia.
- Seizures.

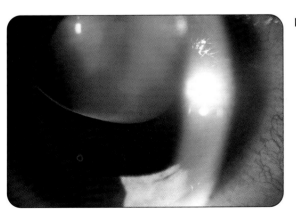

Fig. 1.64

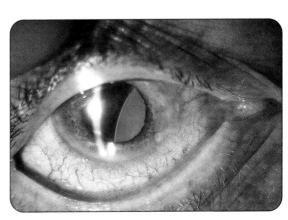

Fig. 1.65

Anterior lenticonus

Signs

- Localized, central, anterior conoid projection of the lens (**Fig. 1.66**).

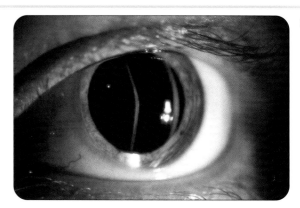

Fig. 1.66

Systemic Association

Alport syndrome

 Look for

- Progressive hemorrhagic nephritis.
- Sensorineural deafness.

Early-onset (presenile) cataract

Systemic Associations

1. Diabetes

- *True diabetic cataract* in young patients is uncommon and is characterized by dense white anterior and posterior subcapsular cortical opacities reminiscent of snowflakes (**Fig. 1.67**).
- *Age-related cataract* may develop earlier and progress quicker (**Fig. 1.68**).

 Look for

- Sensory polyneuropathy involving the feet.
- Accelerated atherosclerosis.
- Skin infections and necrobiosis lipoidica.

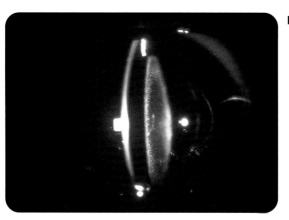

Fig. 1.67

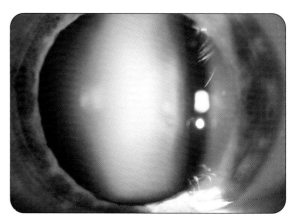

Fig. 1.68

2. Atopic eczema

- Dense, shield-like anterior subcapsular plaque (**Fig. 1.69**).

 Look for

- Dry, erythematous thickening of the skin of the face, side of neck and flexure surfaces.

3. Myotonic dystrophy

- Stellate posterior subcapsular opacity (**Fig. 1.70**).

 Look for

- Mournful facial expression.

- Myotonia of peripheral muscles making release of grip difficult.
- Hypogonadism resulting in infertility and sterility.

4. Neurofibromatosis–2

 Look for

- Bilateral acoustic neuromas.

5. Other

- Cushing syndrome
- Hyperornithinemia.
- Cerebrotendinous xanthomatosis.
- Wilson disease.

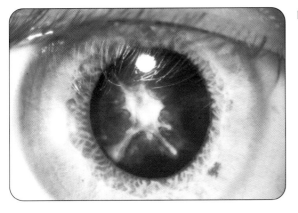

Fig. 1.69

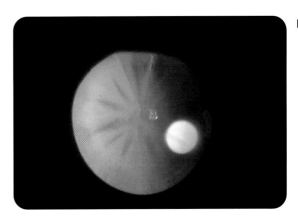

Fig. 1.70

Drug-induced cataract

1. Posterior subcapsular (Fig. 1.71)

 Look for

- Corticosteroids.
- Busulfan.

2. Anterior capsular (Fig. 1.72)

 Look for

- Chlorpromazine.
- Amiodarone.

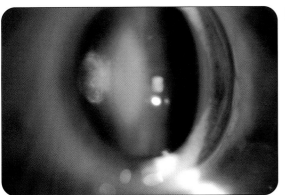

Fig. 1.71

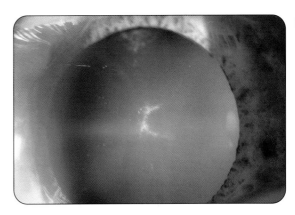

Fig. 1.72

GLAUCOMA

Signs

- Raised intraocular pressure.
- Cupping of the optic nerve head (**Fig. 1.73**).
- Visual field loss.

- Enlarged cornea (buphthalmos) (**Fig. 1.74**) if the intraocular pressure rise occurs prior to the age of three years.

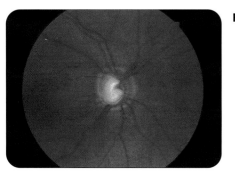

Fig. 1.73

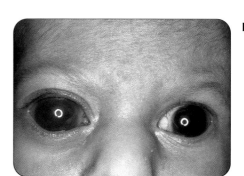

Fig. 1.74

Systemic Associations

1. Struge–Weber syndrome

 Look for

- Leptomeningeal hemangioma.
- Contralateral hemiparesis and hemianopia.
- Epilepsy.

2. Rieger syndrome

 Look for

- Facial and dental anomalies.
- Redundent paraumbilical skin.

3. Waardenburg syndrome

 Look for

- White forelock and premature graying.
- Fusion of eyebrows or an unusual facial hair distribution.
- Deafness.

4. Other
- Marfan syndrome.
- Neurofibromatosis–1.
- Weill–Marchesani syndrome.
- Nevus of Ota.

THE VITREOUS

Intermediate uveitis

Signs

- Vitreous cells, 'cotton-ball' infiltrates and strands, which are frequently bilateral but asymmetrical (**Fig. 1.75**).

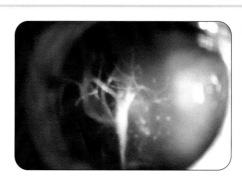

Fig. 1.75

Systemic Associations

1. Sarcoidosis

 Look for

- *Cutaneous lesions* – erythema nodosum, lupus pernio and granulomas.
- *Pulmonary disease* – hilar adenopathy, parenchymal infiltrates and fibrosis.
- *Neurological lesions* – multifocal peripheral neuropathy with a predilection for the facial nerve, meningeal infiltration and CNS granulomata.

2. Multiple sclerosis

 Look for

- *Spinal cord lesions* – weakness, stiffness and sphincter disturbance.
- *Brain stem lesions* – diplopia, nystagmus, dysarthria and dysphagia.
- *Hemisphere lesions* – hemiparesis, hemianopia and dysphasia.

3. Whipple disease

 Look for

- Malabsorption.
- Migratory polyarthritis.
- Pulmonary, cardiac and CNS involvement.

4. Non-Hodgkin large B-cell lymphoma

 Look for

- CNS involvement.

5. Other
- Lyme disease.
- Cat-scratch fever.
- Waldenström macroglobulinemia.

Vitreous opacities

1. Hemorrhage (Fig. 1.76)

 Look for

- *Diabetes* – bleeding from new vessels in proliferative diabetic retinopathy.
- *Hypertension* – bleeding from secondary neovascularization following a branch retinal vein occlusion.
- *Sickle cell disease* – bleeding from new vessels in proliferative sickle-cell retinopathy.

2. Iridescent particles (asteroid hyalosis) (Fig. 1.77)

 Look for

- Diabetes mellitus.

3. Sheet-like ('glass-wool') opacities (Fig. 1.78)

 Look for

- Primary amyloidosis.

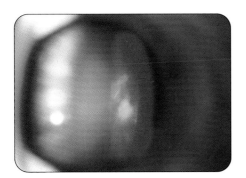

Fig. 1.76

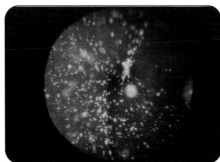

Fig. 1.77

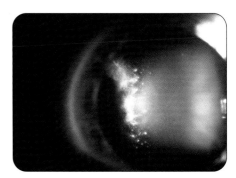

Fig. 1.78

VASCULAR FUNDUS LESIONS

Cotton-wool spots

Signs

- Small, white, superficial lesions with indistinct borders (**Fig. 1.79**). Their presence signifies focal retinal ischemia caused by occlusion of precapillary arterioles.

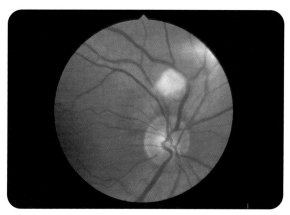

Fig. 1.79

Systemic Associations

1. Diabetes

 Signs

- Preproliferative retinopathy – associated venous abnormalities and deep retinal hemorrhages (**Fig. 1.80**).

 Look for

- Sensory polyneuropathy involving the feet.
- Accelerated atherosclerosis.
- Renal disease.

2. Severe hypertension

 Signs

- Associated flame-shaped hemorrhages (**Fig. 1.81**).

 Look for

- Left ventricular hypertrophy.
- Coronary artery disease and stroke.
- Renal disease.

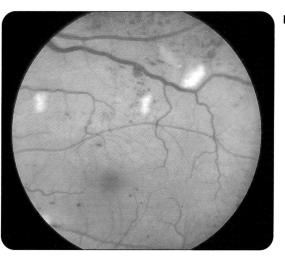

Fig. 1.80

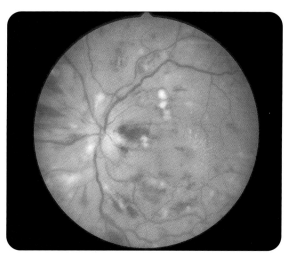

Fig. 1.81

3. AIDS

 Signs

- Variable number of scattered cotton-wool spots (**Fig. 1.82**) which may occasionally be associated with a few retinal hemorrhages.

 Look for

a. *Opportunistic infections* – protozoan, viral, fungal and bacterial.
b. *Tumors* – Kaposi sarcoma and B-cell lymphoma.

4. Antiphospholipid antibody syndrome

 Signs

- Associated venous dilatation.

 Look for

- Recurrent arterial and venous thromboses in a young adult.

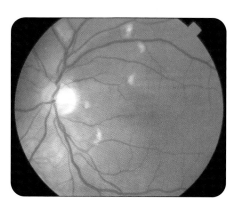

Fig. 1.82

- Recurrent spontaneous abortions.
- Renal disease.

5. Other
- Scleroderma.
- Systemic lupus erythematosus.
- Dermatomyositis.
- Giant cell arteritis.
- Acute pancreatitis.
- Goodpasture syndrome.

Roth spots

Signs

- Flame-shape hemorrhages with pale centers (**Fig. 1.83**).

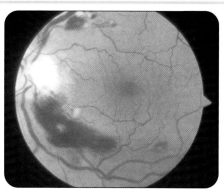

Fig. 1.83

Systemic Associations

1. Severe anemias

 Look for

- Pallor of mucous membranes.

2. Leukemias

 Look for

- Lymphadenopathy and splenomegaly.
- Anemia, purpura and easy bruising.

3. Bacterial endocarditis.

 Look for

- Fever and heart murmurs.
- Splenomegaly.
- Splinter hemorrhages under the nails and Osler nodes.

Hard exudates

Signs

- Yellow, waxy plaques with relatively distinct margins which are most frequently located at the posterior pole.

Systemic Associations

1. Diabetes

 Signs

- Background retinopathy – hard exudates arranged in rings or clumps and associated with microaneurysms and hemorrhages (**Fig. 1.84**).

 Look for

(*see* Cotton-wool spots, p. 34).

2. Severe hypertension

 Signs

- Hard exudates arranged in a star figure at the macular associated with cotton-wool spots (**Fig. 1.85**).

 Look for

(*see* Cotton-wool spots, p. 34)

3. Raised intracranial pressure

 Signs

- Hard exudates associated with disc edema (papilledema) (**Fig. 1.86**).

 Look for

- Cerebral tumor.
- Benign intracranial hypertension.
- Meningitis.

4. Neuroretinitis

 Signs

- Hard exudates arranged in a star figure at the macula (**Fig. 1.87**)

 Look for

- Cat-scratch fever.
- Lyme disease.
- Acquired syphilis.

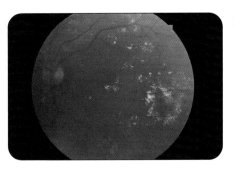

Fig. 1.84

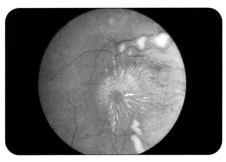

Fig. 1.85

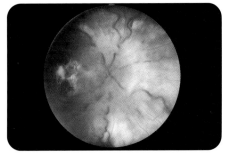

Fig. 1.86

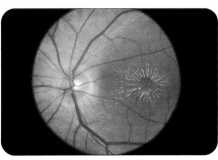

Fig. 1.87

Neovascularization

Signs

- Neovascularization is characterized by the development of new vessels secondary to retinal ischemia.
- The new vessels may be flat or elevated and they may or may not be associated with gliosis.

Systemic Associations

1. New vessels on the disc and/or along the major vascular arcades (Fig. 1.88)

 Look for

- Proliferative diabetic retinopathy.

2. Peripheral new vessels (Fig. 1.89)

 Look for

- Sickle-cell disease.
- Sarcoidosis.
- Chronic myeloid leukemia.

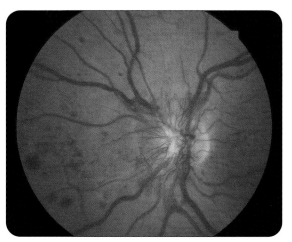

Fig. 1.88

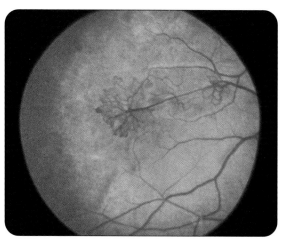

Fig. 1.89

Retinal emboli

1. Fibrinoplatelet

 Signs

- Dull gray, elongated particles which are usually multiple.
- Occasionally they may fill the entire lumen of an arteriole (**Fig. 1.90**).
- May cause amaurosis fugax.

 Look for

- Carotid artery disease.

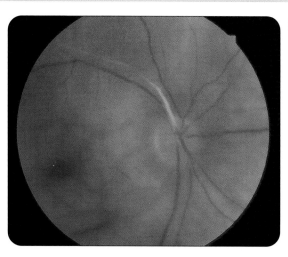

Fig. 1.90

2. Cholesterol (Hollenhorst plaques)

 Signs

- Small, glistening, usually multiple crystals typically located at bifurcations (**Fig. 1.91**)
- They are frequently asymptomatic.

 Look for

- Carotid artery disease.

3. Calcific

 Signs

- White, solitary particle which is most frequently located on or near the optic disc (**Fig. 1.92**).

- May cause permanent arterial occlusion (*see* below).

 Look for

- Cardiac valve or aortic arch calcification.

4. Other
- Mitral valve disease – emboli composed of thrombus.
- Bacterial endocarditis – emboli composed of heart valve vegetations.
- Atrial myxoma – myxomatous emboli.
- Acute pancreatitis – lipid emboli.

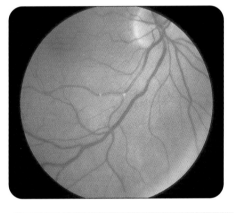

Fig. 1.91

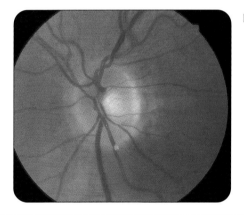

Fig. 1.92

Arterial occlusion

Signs

- Attenuation of arterioles and veins.
- Sludging and segmentation of the blood column.

- White retina in the area supplied by the obstructed artery (**Fig. 1.93**).
- Cherry red spot may be present at the macula if the central retinal artery is occluded.
- A cilioretinal artery, if present, will be spared (**Fig. 1.94**).

Fig. 1.93

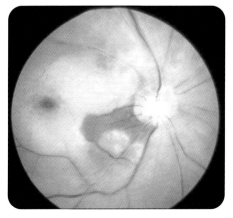

Fig. 1.94

Systemic Associations

1. In the elderly

 Look for

- Hypertension and atherosclerosis.
- Emboli from the carotid artery (*see* above).
- Giant cell arteritis (cilioretinal artery occlusion).

2. In young adults

 Look for

- Hypercoagulation disorders (protein S deficiency, antithrombin III deficiency, 'sticky platelet syndrome' and antiphospholipid antibody syndrome).

- Emboli from abnormal cardiac valves (*see* above).
- Systemic lupus erythematosus.
- Polyarteritis nodosa.
- Sickle-cell disease.
- Hyperhomocystinemia.
- Homocystinuria.
- Migraine.
- Kawasaki syndrome.
- Behçet disease.

Slow-flow retinopathy

Signs

- Venous dilatation, segmentation, and tortuosity associated with hemorrhages (**Fig. 1.95**).

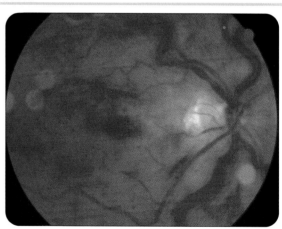

Fig. 1.95

Systemic Associations

 Look for hyperviscosity

- Polycythemia rubra vera.
- Chronic leukemias.
- Waldenström macroglobulinemia.
- Multiple myeloma.

Retinal vein occlusion

Signs

- Venous dilatation, flame-shaped hemorrhages, and cotton-wool spots.
- In branch vein occlusion the changes are confined to one quadrant (**Fig. 1.96**).
- In central vein occlusion they affect all four quadrants (**Fig. 1.97**).

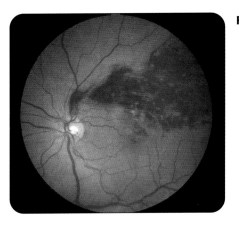

Fig. 1.96

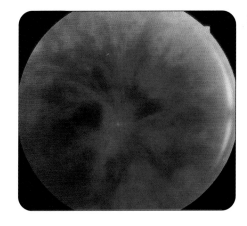

Fig. 1.97

Systemic Associations

 Look for

- Hypertension.
- Diabetes mellitus.
- Hyperlipoproteinemia.

- Antiphospholipid antibody syndrome.
- Hyperviscosity.
- Retinal periphlebitis.

INFLAMMATORY FUNDUS LESIONS

Venous vasculitis (periphlebitis)

Signs

- Initially, patchy, fluffy, white haziness surrounding the venous blood column (**Fig. 1.98**).
- Later venous sheathing.
- If severe, periphlebitis may cause venous occlusion which in turn may result in secondary retinal neovascularization.

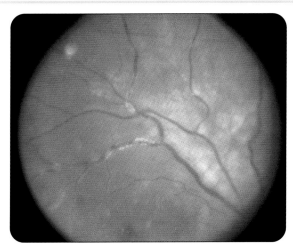

Fig. 1.98

Systemic Associations

1. Sarcoidosis

 Signs

• Rarely, very severe periphlebitis results in perivascular 'candle-wax drippings' (**Fig. 1.99**).

 Look for

• *Cutaneous lesions* – erythema nodosum, lupus pernio and granulomas.
• *Pulmonary disease* – hilar adenopathy, parenchymal infiltrates and fibrosis.
• *Neurological lesions* – cranial nerve palsies, meningeal infiltration and CNS granulomas.

2. Behçet disease

 Signs

• Periphlebitis may be associated with hemorrhage and venous occlusion (**Fig. 1.100**).
• In some cases periarteritis may coexist (*see* below).

 Look for

• Recurrent, painful oral and genital ulceration.
• Cutaneous hypersensitivity, erythema nodosum and acneiform lesions.
• Recurrent thrombophlebitis.

3. AIDS

 Signs

• Periphlebitis which is frequently associated with cytomegalovirus retinitis (**Fig. 1.101**).

 Look for

• *Opportunistic infections* – protozoan, viral, fungal and bacterial.
• *Tumors* – Kaposi sarcoma and B-cell lymphoma.

4. Other
• Multiple sclerosis.
• Tuberculosis.
• Cat-scratch fever.
• Whipple disease.
• Crohn disease.

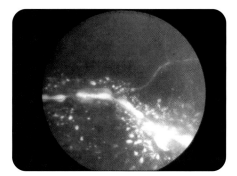

Fig. 1.99

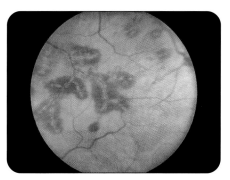

Fig. 1.100

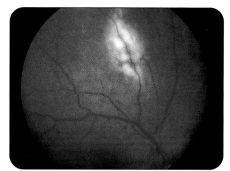

Fig. 1.101

Arterial vasculitis (periarteritis)

Signs

• Initially, patchy, fluffy white haziness surrounding the arteriolar blood column.
• Later arteriolar sheathing.
• Severe periarteritis may result in multiple branch artery occlusions (**Fig. 1.102**).

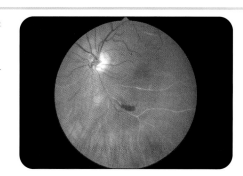

Fig. 1.102

Systemic Associations

1. Sarcoidosis

 Signs

- Usually multifocal choroiditis (**Fig. 1.110**).

 Look for

(*see* Periphlebitis, p. 40)

2. AIDS

- *Cryptococcal choroiditis* – multifocal choroiditis.
- *Pneumocystis carinii choroiditis* – multifocal choroiditis (**Fig. 1.111**).

 Look for

(*see* Periphlebitis, p. 40)

3. Histoplasmosis

 Signs

- Multifocal atrophic 'histo spots' (**Fig. 1.112**).
- Associated with peripapillary atrophy, peripheral linear atrophic streaks and occasionally choroidal neovascularization at the macula.
- Vitritis is absent.

 Look for

- Usually no systemic features.
- Occasionally malaise, cough and hilar lymphadenopathy.

4. Harada disease

 Signs

- Initially multifocal choroiditis (**Fig. 1.113**).
- Later exudative retinal detachment.

 Look for

- Headache and neck stiffness.
- Tinnitus, vertigo and deafness.
- Convulsions, cranial nerve palsies and paresis.

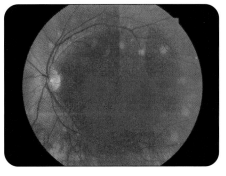

Fig. 1.110

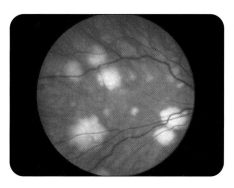

Fig. 1.111

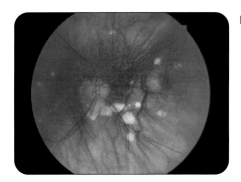

Fig. 1.112

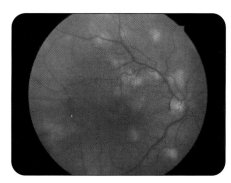

Fig. 1.113

5. Tuberculosis

 Signs

- Usually multifocal choroiditis (**Fig. 1.114**).

 Look for

- Constitutional symptoms.
- Pulmonary symptoms.

6. Other
- Acquired syphilis.
- Coccidioidomycosis.
- Onchocerciasis.

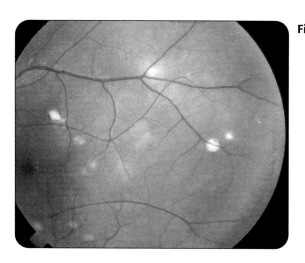

Fig. 1.114

DYSTROPHIC FUNDUS LESIONS

Pigmentary retinopathy

Signs

- Classical retinitis pigmentosa is characterized by bilateral, peripheral, bone spicule perivascular pigmentation, arteriolar narrowing and waxy disc pallor (**Figs 1.115** and **1.116**).

- Frequently, however, the above signs may be atypical (**Fig. 1.117**) or not all present (**Fig. 1.118**).

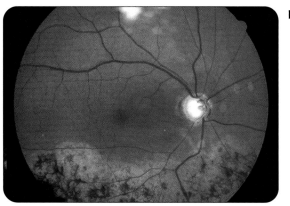

Fig. 1.115

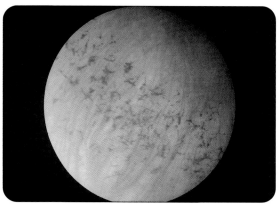

Fig. 1.116

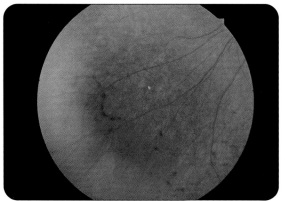

Fig. 1.117

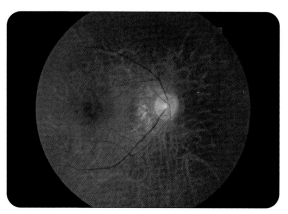

Fig. 1.118

Systemic Associations

1. Bassen–Kornzweig syndrome

 Look for

- Ptosis and progressive external ophthalmoplegia.
- Steatorrhea and malabsorption.
- Spinocerobellar ataxia.

2. Kearns–Sayre syndrome

 Look for

- Ptosis and progressive external ophthalmoplegia.
- Heart block.
- Ataxia and proximal limb weakness.

3. Refsum syndrome

 Look for

- Mixed motor and sensory polyneuropathy.
- Cerebellar ataxia, deafness and anosmia.
- Ichthyosis.

4. Usher syndrome

 Look for

- Deafness.

5. Friedreich ataxia

 Look for

- Spinocerebellar degeneration in childhood.
- Gait ataxia and deformity of feet.
- Cardiomyopathy and deafness.

6. Myotonic dystrophy

 Look for

- Mournful facial expression and ptosis.
- Myotonia of peripheral muscles making release of grip difficult.
- Hypogonadism resulting in infertility or sterility.

7. Cystinosis types 1 and 3

 Look for

- Blond hair and fair complexion (type 1).
- Renal disease (types 1 and 3).

Albinoid fundus

Signs

- Diffuse lack of fundus pigment with unmasking of choroidal vessels (**Fig. 1.119**).

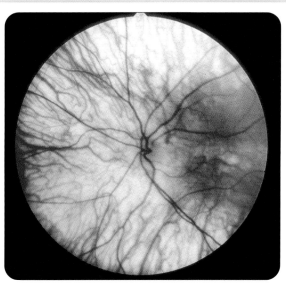

Fig. 1.119

Systemic Associations

1. Oculocutaneous albinism

 Look for

- Photophobia.
- White hair and pink skin.
- Absence of pigmented skin nevi.

2. Chédiak–Higashi syndrome

 Look for

- Recurrent pyogenic infections.
- Hepatomegaly.
- Lymphadenopathy.

3. Hermansky–Pudlak syndrome

 Look for

- Easy brusing, especially after aspirin ingestion.
- Pulmonary fibrosis.

4. Waardenburg syndrome

 Look for

- Heterochromia iridis.
- Fusion of eyebrows and unusual facial hair distribution.
- Deafness.

Gyrate atrophy of the retina and choroid

Signs

- Circular patches of peripheral chorioretinal atrophy with scalloped borders (**Fig. 1.120**).

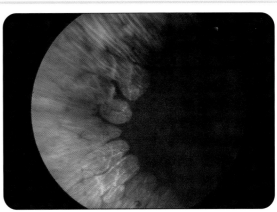

Fig. 1.120

Systemic Association

Hyperornithinemia

 Look for

- Ornithinuria.

Angioid streaks

Signs

- Linear gray or dark-red lesions with irregular serrated edges lying beneath normal retinal blood vessels (**Fig. 1.121**).
- The streaks intercommunicate around the disc and then radiate outwards.

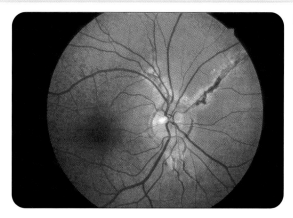

Fig. 1.121

Systemic Associations

1. Pseudoxanthoma elasticum (Grönblad–Strandberg syndrome)

 Look for

- Characteristic skin lesions.
- Accelerated atherosclerosis.
- Floppy mitral valve.

2. Ehlers–Danlos syndrome type 6

 Look for

- Thin and hyperelastic skin which bruises easily and heals slowly.

- Joint hyperextensibility and easy dislocation.
- Dissecting aortic aneurysm and mitral valve disease.

3. Paget disease

 Look for

- Bony enlargement, deformity and warmth.
- Deafness.

4. Other
- Hemoglobinopathies.
- Acromegaly.

Crystalline maculopathy

Signs

- Multitude of glistening crystals at the posterior pole (**Fig. 1.122**).

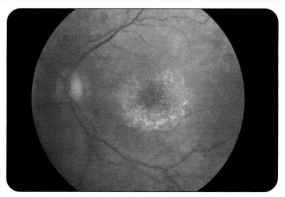

Fig. 1.122

Systemic Associations

1. Tamoxifen toxicity

 Look for

- Breast carcinoma or a strong family history of the disease.

2. Oxalosis

 Look for

- Heart disease.
- Renal disease.

INTRAOCULAR TUMORS

Benign tumors

1. Congenital hypertrophy of the retinal pigment epithelium

 Signs

- Multiple, frequently bilateral, fishtail-shaped pigmented lesions (**Fig. 1.123**).

 Look for

- Gardner syndrome.
- Turcot syndrome.

2. Choroidal nevus

 Signs

- Flat or minimally elevated, oval, slate-gray lesion which is frequently associated with surface drusen (**Fig. 1.124**).

 Look for

- Neurofibromatosis–1 (multiple and bilateral nevi).

3. Combined hamartoma of the retinal pigment epithelium and retina

 Signs

- Solitary, unilateral, elevated lesion associated with variable gliosis, capillary dilatation and vascular tortuosity (**Fig. 1.125**).

 Look for

- Neurofibromatosis–2.

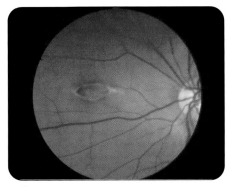

Fig. 1.123

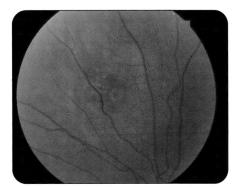

Fig. 1.124

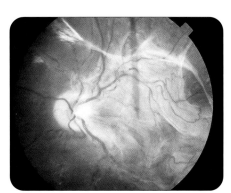

Fig. 1.125

4. Retinal capillary hemangioma

 Signs

- Orange–red mass associated with dilated and tortuous supplying artery and draining vein (**Fig. 1.126**).
- The tumor is usually peripheral but may sometimes be located on or near the disc (**Fig. 1.127**).
- Macular hard exudates may develop.

 Look for

- von Hippel–Lindau syndrome (usually multiple and may be bilateral).

5. Diffuse choroidal hemangioma

 Signs

- Unilateral, thickening of the choroid at the posterior pole which has a deep red color (**Fig. 1.128**).

 Look for

- Sturge–Weber syndrome.

6. Retinal astrocytoma

 Signs

- A white nodular lesion which my have a mulberry-like appearance (**Fig. 1.129**).

 Look for

- Tuberous sclerosis (may be multiple and bilateral).
- Neurofibromatosis–1.

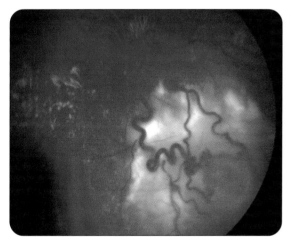

Fig. 1.126

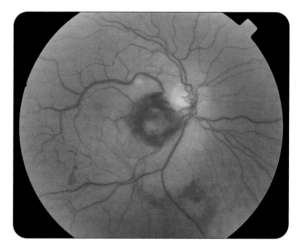

Fig. 1.127

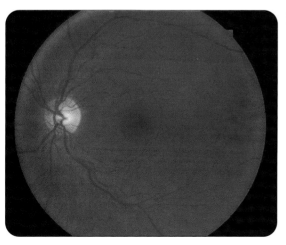

Fig. 1.128

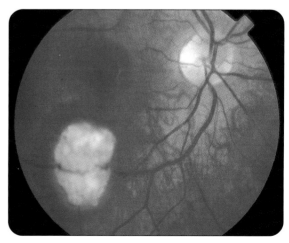

Fig. 1.129

Malignant tumors

1. Choroidal metastatic carcinoma

 Signs

- Fast-growing, creamy-white, placoid or oval lesion most frequently located at the posterior pole (**Fig. 1.130**).
- The deposits may be solitary, multiple or bilateral.
- Secondary exudative retinal detachement is common.

 Look for

- Most frequently bronchial or breast carcinoma.
- Less frequently carcinoma of the kidney, testis and gastrointestinal tract.

2. Choroidal melanoma

 Signs

- Solitary, unilateral, elevated oval-shaped mass (**Fig. 1.131**).

 Look for

- Nevus of Ota.

3. Intraocular lymphoma

 Signs

- Multiple, oval, yellowish subretinal infiltrates with indistinct borders (**Fig. 1.132**).
- Occasionally the infiltrates coalesce (**Fig. 1.133**).

 Look for

- CNS non-Hodgkin B-cell lymphoma.

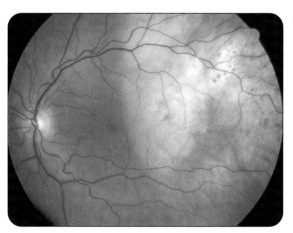

Fig. 1.130

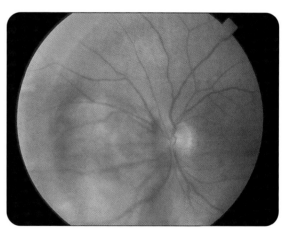

Fig. 1.131

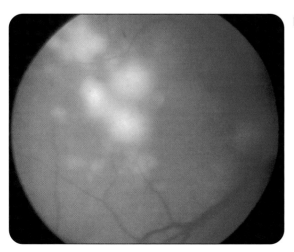

Fig. 1.132

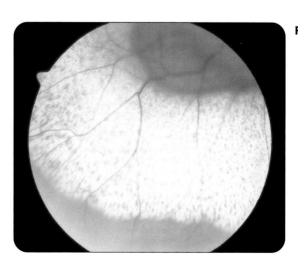

Fig. 1.133

THE OPTIC NERVE

Primary optic atrophy

Signs

- White, flat optic disc with a clearly delineated outline (**Fig. 1.134**).
- Reduction in the number of small blood vessels crossing the disc.

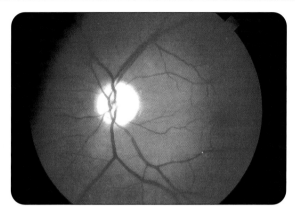

Fig. 1.134

Systemic Associations

1. Following optic neuritis

 Look for

- Multiple sclerosis.
- Devic disease.
- Schilder disease.

2. Following compression

 Look for

- Paget disease.

- Acromegaly (acidophil pituitary adenoma).
- Cushing disease (basophil pituitary adenoma).
- Neurofibromatosis–1 (optic nerve glioma).

3. Other
- Pernicious anemia.
- Charcot–Marie–Tooth disease.
- Friedreich ataxia.

Anterior ischemic optic neuropathy

Signs

- Disc pallor and edema (**Fig. 1.135**) which is frequently associated with small splinter-shaped peripapillary hemorrhages.

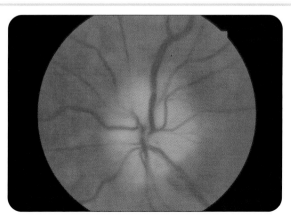

Fig. 1.135

Systemic Associations

1. Giant cell arteritis

 Look for

- Jaw claudication, anorexia and neck pain.
- Scalp tenderness and thickened temporal arteries.
- Polymyalgia rheumatica.

2. Hypertension

 Look for

- Left vertricular hypertrophy.
- Coronary artery disease and stroke.
- Renal disease.

3. Systemic lupus erythematosus

 Look for

- Facial rash with a characteristic 'butterfly' distribution.
- Cutaneous vasculitis and photosensitivity.
- Glomerulonephritis.

4. Antiphospholipid antibody syndrome

 Look for

- Recurrent arterial and venous thromboses in a young adult.
- Recurrent spontaneous abortions.
- Renal disease.

Papillitis

Signs

- Disc hyperemia and edema (**Fig. 1.136**) which may be associated with disc hemorrhages and cells in the vitreous.

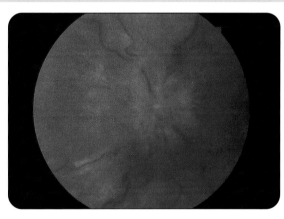

Fig. 1.136

Systemic Associations

1. Childhood viral infections (frequently bilateral).

2. Demyelinating diseases
- Usually cause retrobulbar neuritis and rarely papillitis.

Neuroretinitis

Signs

- Papillitis associated with a macular star and occasionally juxtapapillary exudates (**Fig. 1.137**).

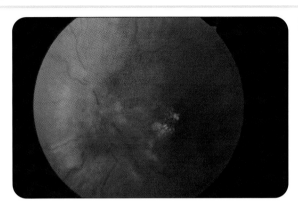

Fig. 1.137

Systemic Associations

1. Cat-scratch fever.

 Look for

- Fever and malaise.
- Skin pustule and regional lymphadenophathy.

2. Lyme disease stage 2

 Look for

- Cardiac dysrhythmia and myocarditis.
- Arthralgia.
- Neuropathy.

3. Other
- Viral infections.
- Acquired syphilis.

Bilateral disc swelling

Systemic Associations

1. Raised intracranial pressure (papilledema)

 Signs

a. *Early* (**Fig. 1.138**)
- Mildly elevated discs, slight hyperemia, and indistinct margins.

b. *Established* (**Fig. 1.139**)
- Moderately elevated discs, severe hyperemia, and edema.
- Associated flame-shaped hemorrhages and cotton-wool spots.

c. *Chronic* (**Fig. 1.140**)
- Very severely elevated discs but without hemorrhages and cotton-wool spots.

d. *Atrophic* (**Fig. 1.141**)
- White, slightly elevated discs with indistinct margins.

 Look for

- Cerebral tumor.
- Benign intracranial hypertension.
- Meningitis.

2. Malignant hypertension

 Signs

- Severe elevated discs with flame-shaped hemorrhages, cotton-wool spots and a macular star (**Fig. 1.142**).
- Associated other hypertensive vascular changes.

3. Other

- Bilateral diabetic papillopathy.
- Bilateral compressive thyroid optic neuropathy.
- Bilateral papillitis.
- Bilateral simultaneous anterior ischemic optic neuropathy.

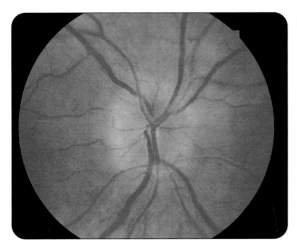

Fig. 1.138

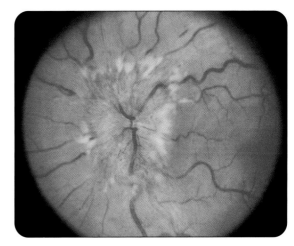

Fig. 1.139

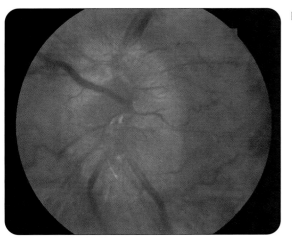

Fig. 1.140

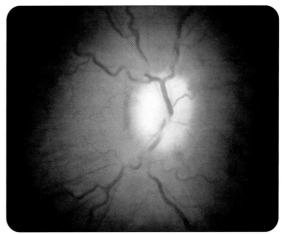

Fig. 1.141

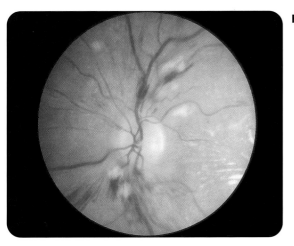

Fig. 1.142

OPTHALMOPLEGIA

Neurological palsies

Signs

1. Third nerve palsy (left)
- Ptosis and limitation of adduction (**Fig. 1.143a**).
- Limitation of elevation (**Fig. 1.143b**).
- Limitation of depression (**Fig. 1.143c**).
- Normal abduction (**Fig. 1.143d**).
- Internal opthalmoplegia involving the pupil is usually present if the cause is an aneurysm or a tumor.
- Paralysis of accommodation.

2. Fourth nerve palsy (right)
- Right eye is higher (hypertropia) then the left in the primary position.
- Limitation of right depression in adduction with vertical diplopia (**Fig. 1.144a**).
- Right overaction on left gaze (**Fig. 1.144b**).

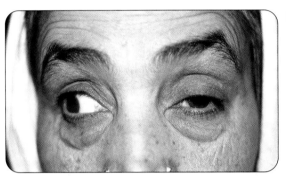

Fig. 1.143a

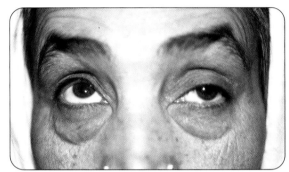

Fig. 1.143b

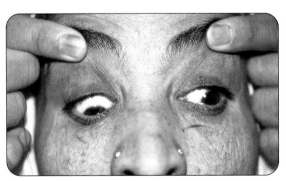

Fig. 1.143c

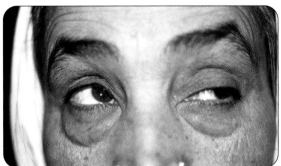

Fig. 1.143d

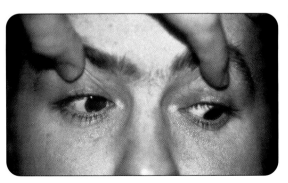

Fig. 1.144a

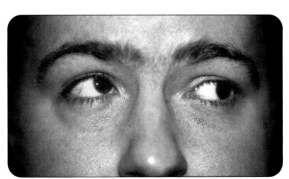

Fig. 1.144b

3. Sixth nerve palsy (left)

- Left limitation on left gaze with horizontal diplopia (**Fig. 1.145a**).

- Normal left adduction (**Fig. 1.145b**).

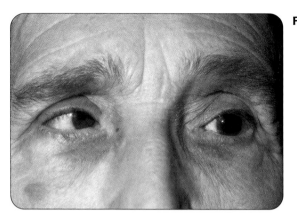

Fig. 1.145a

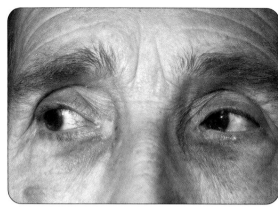

Fig. 1.145b

Systemic Associations

1. **Diabetes**

2. **Hypertension**

3. **Aneurysm**

4. **Trauma**

5. **Cerebral tumor**

6. **Benign intracranial hypertension**

7. **Demyelination**

8. **Other**
   - Carotid-cavernous fistula.
   - Sarcoidosis.
   - Giant cell arteritis.
   - Systemic lupus erythematosus.
   - Paget disease.
   - Lyme disease.
   - Wernicke encephalopathy.

Individual myopathic palsies

Signs

- Restriction of individual muscles (**Fig. 1.146**).

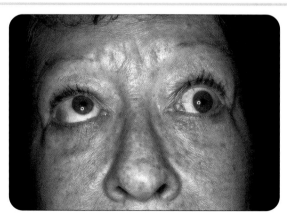

Fig. 1.146

Tumors
Cerebral metastases
Tuberous sclerosis
Sturge–Weber syndrome
von Hippel–Lindau syndrome
Neurofibromatosis–1
Neurofibromatosis–2
Acromegaly
Cushing disease

Deafness
Paget disease
Usher syndrome
Harada disease
Cogan syndrome
Relapsing polychondritis
Neurofibromatosis–2
Waardenburg syndrome
Other

Mental retardation
Down syndrome
Homocystinuria
Tuberous sclerosis
Weill–Marchesani syndrome
Hyperlysinemia
Sturge–Weber syndrome

Mental deterioration
Cerebrotendinous xanthomatosis
Myxedema
Progressive supranuclear ophthalmoplegia
(Steele–Richardson–Olszewski syndrome)
Wernicke encephalopathy
Xeroderma pigmentosum
Wilson disease

THE FACE

Facial rashes and pigmentary changes

Systemic Associations

1. Atopic eczema

 Signs

- Dry, itchy, erythematous thickening of facial skin (**Fig. 2.1**).

 Look for

- Chronic keratoconjunctivitis (vernal or atopic).
- Early-onset cataract.

2. Rosacea

 Signs

- Erythema and papules on the glabella, cheeks, nose and chin (**Fig. 2.2**).

 Look for

- Inferior peripheral corneal infiltration, vascularization and thinning.

3. Sarcoidosis

 Signs

- Violaceous lesions with a predilection for the nose (lupus pernio) (**Fig. 2.3**).

 Look for

- Keratoconjunctivitis sicca.
- Anterior uveitis.
- Retinal periphlebitis and multifocal choroiditis.

4. Systemic lupus erythematosus

 Signs

- Erythematous rash involving the cheeks and bridge of the nose in a 'butterfly' distribution (**Fig. 2.4**).

 Look for

- Keratoconjunctivitis sicca.
- Peripheral ulcerative keratitis.
- Retinal periarteritis.

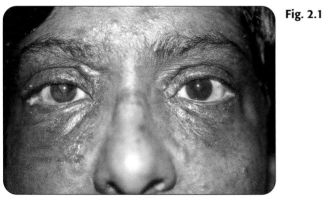
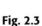
Fig. 2.1

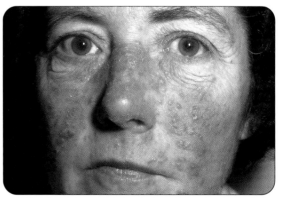
Fig. 2.2

Fig. 2.3

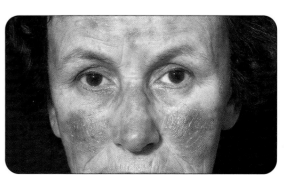
Fig. 2.4

5. Dermatomyositis

 Signs

- Extensive erythematous rash (**Fig. 2.5**).

 Look for

- Keratoconjunctivis sicca.
- Scleritis.
- Retinal cotton-wool spots.

6. Sturge–Weber syndrome

 Signs

- Port-wine stain (nevus flammeus) which is a sharply demarcated, soft, purple patch which does not blanch with pressure.
- The lesion may be localized or it may be extensive and involve the distribution of the first and second divisions of the trigeminal nerve (**Fig. 2.6**).
- Both sides of the face are occasionally involved.

 Look for

- Ipsilateral glaucoma.
- Ipsilateral diffuse choroidal hemangioma.

7. Tuberous sclerosis

 Signs

- Red papules on the cheeks and nose consisting of angiofibromas (adenoma sebaceum) (**Fig. 2.7**).

 Look for

- Retinal or optic disc astrocytomas which may be bilateral and multiple.

8. Xeroderma pigmentosum

 Signs

- Bird-like facies.
- Atrophic, scaling and pigmentary skin changes (**Fig. 2.8**).
- Propensity to skin malignancies.

 Look for

- Conjunctival cicatrization.
- Keratitis.

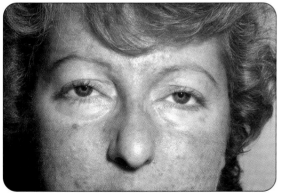

Fig. 2.5

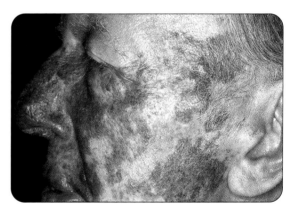

Fig. 2.6

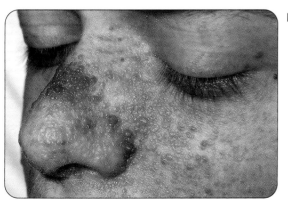

Fig. 2.7

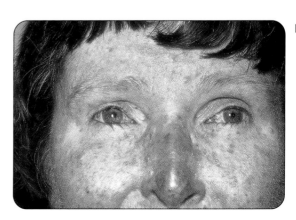

Fig. 2.8

9. Nevus of Ota

 Signs

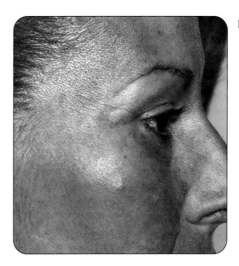
Fig. 2.9

- Unilateral hyperpigmentation of deep facial skin, most frequently in the distribution of the first and second divisions of the trigeminal nerve (**Fig. 2.9**).

 Look for

- Ipsilateral episcleral and uveal hyperpigmentation.
- Melanoma of the uvea, orbit and optic nerve.

Blond hair and fair complexion

Systemic Associations

1. Oculocutaneous albinism (Fig. 2.10)

 Look for

- Iris transillumination.
- Fundus hypopigmentation.

2. Homocystinuria (Fig. 2.11)

 Look for

- Downward lens subluxation.
- Myopia and retinal detachment.

3. Infantile nephropathic cystinosis type 1

 Look for

- Corneal crystals.
- Retinopathy.

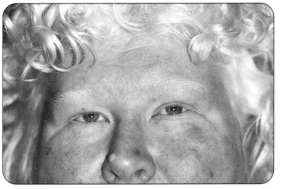
Fig. 2.10

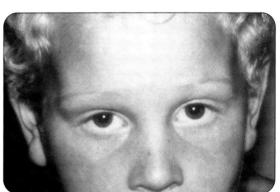
Fig. 2.11

Lack of facial expression

Systemic Associations

1. Myotonic dystrophy

 Signs

- Bilateral facial wasting with hollow cheeks, sagging jaw and variable ptosis (**Fig. 2.12**).

 Look for

- Posterior stellate cataracts.
- Light-near dissociation of pupillary reactions.

2. Myasthenia gravis

 Signs

- Myasthenic involvement of facial muscles and ptosis (**Fig. 2.13**).

 Look for

- Vertical diplopia.

3. Systemic sclerosis

 Signs

- Tight facial skin due to subcutaneous fibrotic changes (**Fig. 2.14**).

 Look for

- Keratoconjunctivitis sicca.
- Retinal cotton-wool spots and hemorrhages.

4. Meretoja syndrome

 Signs

- Facial diplegia (**Fig. 2.15**).

 Look for

- Lattice corneal dystrophy type 2.

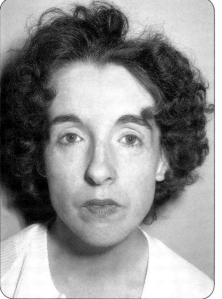

Fig. 2.12

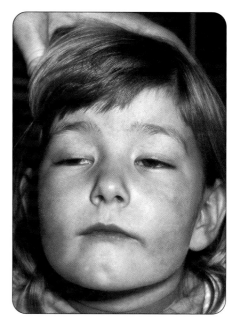

Fig. 2.13

68

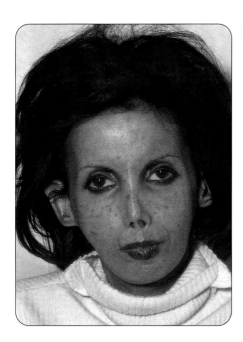

Fig. 2.14

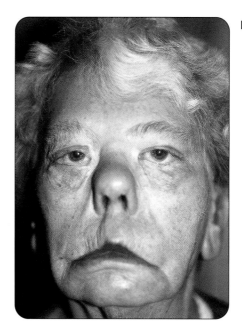

Fig. 2.15

Saddle-shaped nose

Systemic Associations

1. Congenital syphilis

 Cause

- Osteitis of the nasal bone (**Fig. 2.16**).

 Look for

- Interstitial keratitis.
- Pigmentary retinopathy.

2. Wegener granulomatosis

 Cause

- Necrotizing granulomatous vasculitis involving the nose.

 Look for

- Orbital involvement.
- Peripheral ulcerative keratitis.
- Anterior scleritis.

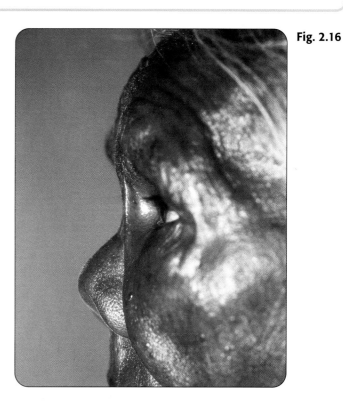

Fig. 2.16

3. Relapsing polychondritis

 Cause

- Recurrent inflammatory swelling, destruction and collapse of the nasal cartilage.

 Look for

- Keratoconjunctivitis sicca.
- Peripheral ulcerative keratitis.
- Anterior scleritis.

4. Leprosy

 Cause

- Destruction of the nasal cartilage and bone (**Fig. 2.17**).

 Look for

- Madarosis.
- Anterior uveitis.
- Keratitis.

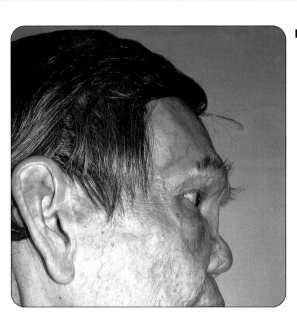

Fig. 2.17

THE MOUTH

Ulceration of mucosa

1. Behçet disease

 Signs

- Recurrent, painful aphthous stomatitis which may involve the buccal mucosa and the tongue (**Fig. 2.18**).

 Look for

- Hypopyon anterior uveitis.
- Retinitis.
- Retinal vasculitis.

2. Reiter syndrome

 Signs

- Transient, painless ulceration (**Fig. 2.19**).

 Look for

- Conjunctivitis.
- Acute anterior uveitis.

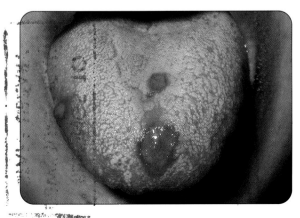

Fig. 2.18

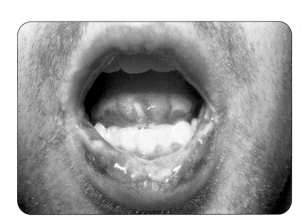

Fig. 2.19

3. Stevens–Johnson syndrome

 Signs

• Mucosal bullae and erosions associated with hemorrhagic crusting of the lips (**Fig. 2.20**).

 Look for

• Initially, subacute membranous conjunctivitis.
• Later variable conjunctival cicatrization.

4. Cicatricial pemphigoid

 Signs

• Mucosal blisters and superficial erosions (**Fig. 2.21**).

 Look for

• Cicatrizing conjunctivitis.

5. Pemphigus vulgaris

 Signs

• Mucosal blisters and erosions (**Fig. 2.22**).

 Look for

• Conjunctivitis.

6. Crohn disease

 Signs

• Aphthous ulceration and glossitis (**Fig. 2.23**).

7. Other
• Ulcerative colitis.
• Epidermolysis bullosa.
• Systemic lupus erythematosus.

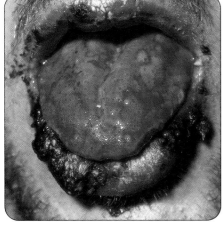

Fig. 2.20

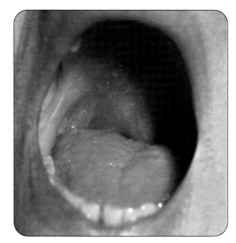

Fig. 2.21

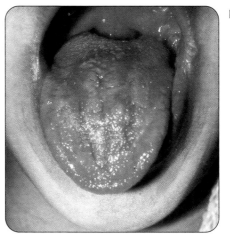

Fig. 2.22

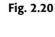

Fig. 2.23

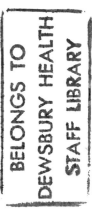

Abnormal dentition

Systemic Associations

1. Congenital syphilis

 Signs

- Mulberry molars and malformed incisors (Hutchinson teeth) (**Fig. 2.24**).

 Look for

- Interstitial keratitis.
- Pigmentary retinopathy.

2. Osteogenesis imperfecta type 3

 Signs

- Small teeth (dentiogenesis imperfecta) (**Fig. 2.25**).

 Look for

- Blue sclera.

3. Rieger syndrome

 Signs

- Small teeth which are also fewer in number (**Fig. 2.26**).

 Look for

- Posterior embryotoxon and iris anomalies.
- Glaucoma.

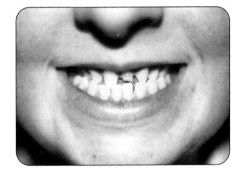

Fig. 2.24

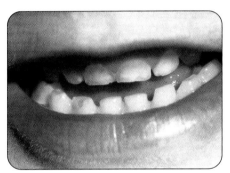

Fig. 2.25

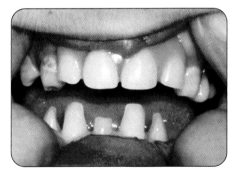

Fig. 2.26

High-arched palate

Systemic Associations

1. Marfan syndrome

 Look for

- Upward lens subluxation.
- Megalocornea and keratoconus.
- Retinal detachment.

2. Pseudoxanthoma elasticum–dominant type 2

Look for

- Blue sclera.
- Mild angioid streaks.

3. Other
- Congenital syphilis.
- Homocystinuria.

Abnormal tongue

Systemic Associations

1. Sjögren syndrome

 Signs

- Dry mouth and tongue (**Fig. 2.27**).

 Look for

- Keratoconjunctivitis sicca.

2. Iron deficiency anemia

 Signs

- Atrophic glossitis with loss of lingual papillae (**Fig. 2.28**).

 Look for

- Flame-shaped retinal hemorrhages, Roth spots, cotton-wool spots and venous tortuosity.

3. Acromegaly

 Signs

- Large tongue (**Fig. 2.29**).

 Look for

- Biltemporal hemianopia.
- Optic atrophy.

4. Endocrine neoplasia type IIb

 Signs

- Thickening of the tongue due to a mucosal neuroma (**Fig. 2.30**).

 Look for

- Eyelid neurofibromas.
- Prominent corneal nerves.

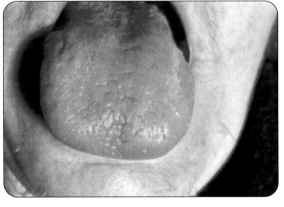

Fig. 2.27

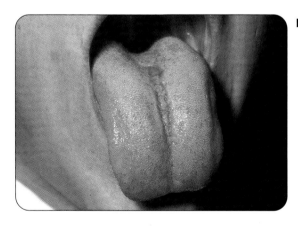

Fig. 2.28

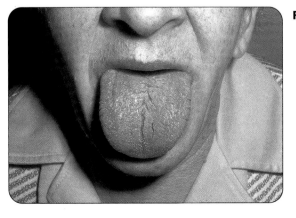

Fig. 2.29

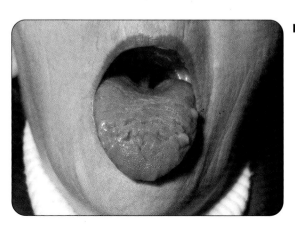

Fig. 2.30

5. Rendu–Osler–Weber syndrome

 Signs

- Telangiectasia of the tongue (**Fig. 2.31**).

 Look for

- Conjunctival telangiectasia.
- Retinal hemorrhages.

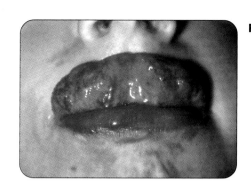

Fig. 2.31

Enlarged parotid glands

Systemic Associations

1. Sarcoidosis (Fig. 2.32).

 Look for

- Heerfordt syndrome – fever, parotid enlargement and uveitis.

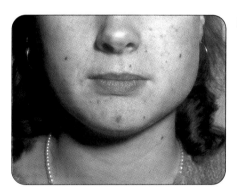

Fig. 2.32

2. Sjögren syndrome (Fig. 2.33).

 Look for

- Keratoconjunctivitis sicca, xerostomia and a connective tissue disease.

3. Lymphoma (Fig. 2.34)

 Look for

- Mikulicz syndrome – lacrimal and salivary gland enlargement.

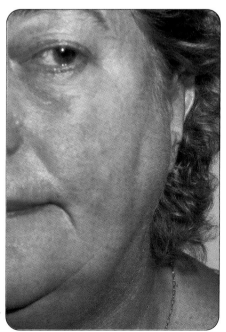

Fig. 2.33

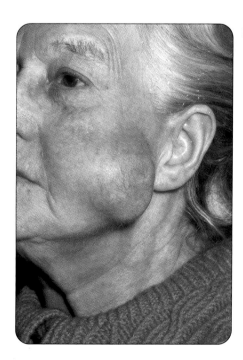

Fig. 2.34

THE SKULL

Lytic bony lesions

1. Metastatic carcinoma (Fig. 2.35).

- Most frequently from breast, bronchus and prostate.

 Look for

- Orbital metastases.
- Choroidal metastases (not prostate).
- Cancer-associated retinopathy.

2. Multiple myeloma (Fig. 2.36).

 Look for

- Corneal crystals.
- Slow-flow retinopathy.

3. Hand–Schüller–Christian disease (Fig. 2.37).

 Look for

- Proptosis.

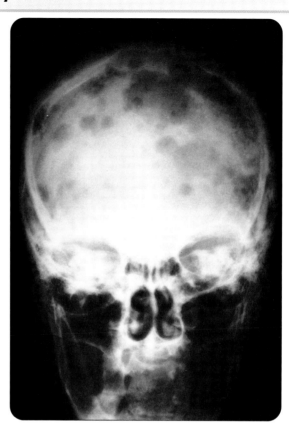

Fig. 2.35

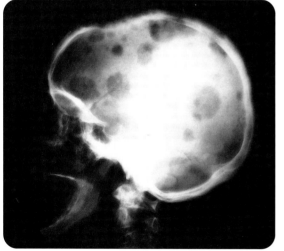

Fig. 2.36

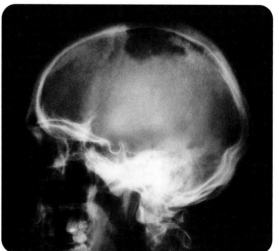

Fig. 2.37

Enlargement

Systemic Associations

1. Paget disease (Fig. 2.38)

 Look for

- Optic atrophy.
- Proptosis.
- Angioid streaks.

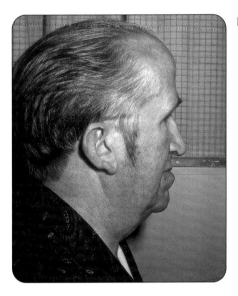

Fig. 2.38

2. Acromegaly (Fig. 2.39)

 Look for

- Bitemporal hemianopia.
- Optic atrophy.
- Angioid streaks.

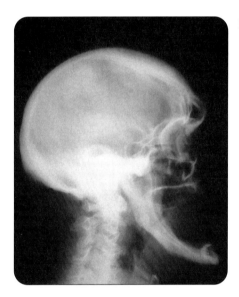

Fig. 2.39

THE NECK

Lymphadenopathy

Signs

- Enlargement of lymph nodes in the neck (**Fig. 2.40**) which may be associated with lymphadenopathy elsewhere and splenomegaly.

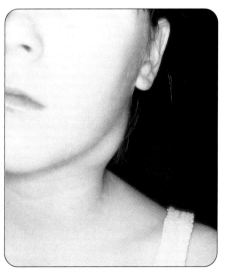

Fig. 2.40

Systemic Associations

1. Lymphoma

 Look for

- Mikulicz syndrome.
- Orbital and conjunctival involvement.
- Uveal infiltration.

2. Leukemia

 Look for

- Orbital involvement in children.
- Pseudo-hypopyon and spontaneous hyphema.
- Retinal hemorrhages and Roth spots.

3. Waldenström macroglobulinemia

 Look for

- Slow-flow retinopathy.
- Cotton-wool spots.
- Corneal crystals.

4. Other

- Sarcoidosis.
- Secondary syphilis.
- Cat-scratch fever.
- Kawasaki disease.
- AIDS.
- Chancroid.
- Systemic lupus erythematosus.
- Whipple disease.

THE HANDS

Long fingers (arachnodactyly)

Systemic Associations

1. Marfan syndrome (Fig. 2.41).

 Look for

- Upward lens subluxation.
- Retinal detachment.

2. Homocystinuria

 Look for

- Downward lens subluxation.
- Myopia and retinal detachment.

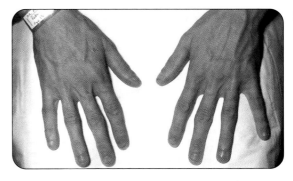

Fig. 2.41

Short fingers (brachydactyly)

Systemic Associations

1. Weill–Marchesani syndrome (Fig. 2.42).

 Look for

- Microspherophakia and lens subluxation.

2. Down syndrome (Fig. 2.43).

Look for

- Brushfield iris spots.
- Keratoconus and blue dot lens opacities.

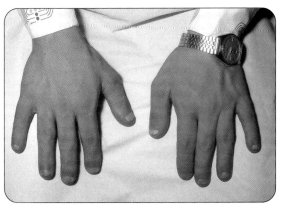

Fig. 2.42

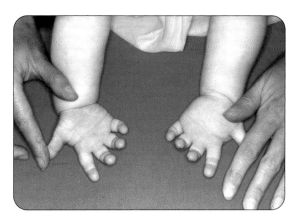

Fig. 2.43

Wasting of small muscles

Systemic Associations

1. Syringomyelia (Fig. 2.44).

 Look for

- Horner syndrome.

2. Charcot–Marie–Tooth disease (Fig. 2.45).

 Look for

- Optic atrophy.

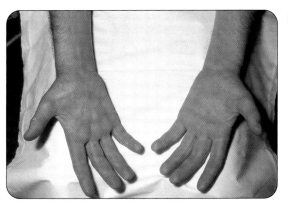

Fig. 2.44

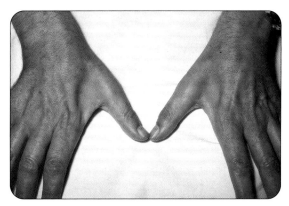

Fig. 2.45

3. Bronchial carcinoma (Fig. 2.46).

 Look for

- Horner syndrome (Pancoat tumor).
- Orbital or choroidal metastases.
- Cancer-related retinopathy.

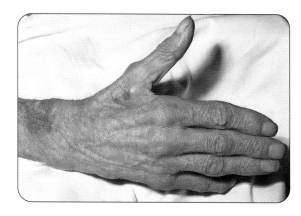

Fig. 2.46

Finger clubbing

Signs

- Increased nail curvature and swelling of the terminal phalanges.

Systemic Associations

1. Bronchial carcinoma (Fig. 2.47).

 Look for

(*see* Wasting of small muscles, above).

2. Thyroid disease (acropachy) (Fig. 2.48).

 Look for

- *Soft tissue signs* – periorbital swelling, chemosis and superior limbic keratoconjunctivitis.

- *Eyelid signs* – lid retraction and lid lag in downgaze.
- *Proptosis* – unilateral or bilateral.
- *Restrictive myopathy* – most frequently involving elevation.
- *Optic neuropathy*.

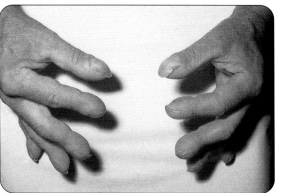

Fig. 2.47

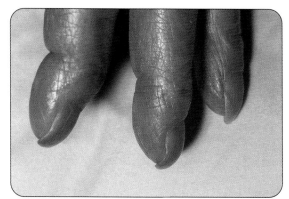

Fig. 2.48

3. Bacterial endocarditis (Fig. 2.49).

 Look for

- Roth spots.
- Retinal artery occlusion.

4. Crohn disease

 Look for

- Acute anterior uveitis.
- Conjunctivitis.

5. Ulcerative colitis

 Look for

- Acute anterior uveitis.

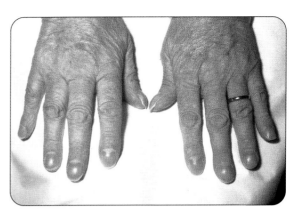

Fig. 2.49

6. Whipple disease

 Look for

- Intermediate uveitis.
- Retinal periphlebitis.

Raynaud phenomenon

Signs

- Intermittent, bilateral vasospasm following exposure to cold.
- The fingers and occasionally the toes become pale, then blue (**Fig. 2.50**), and finally red as the attack passes.

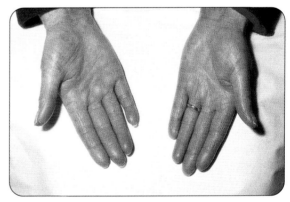

Fig. 2.50

Systemic Associations

1. Scleroderma

 Look for

- Keratoconjunctivitis sicca.
- Retinal cotton-wool spots and hemorrhages.

2. Rheumatoid arthritis

 Look for

- Keratoconjunctivitis sicca.
- Anterior scleritis.
- Peripheral ulcerative kertitis.

3. Systemic lupus erythematosus

 Look for

- Keratoconjunctivitis sicca.
- Peripheral corneal thinning.
- Retinal periarteritis.

4. Dermatomyositis

 Look for

- Keratoconjunctivitis sicca.
- Scleritis.
- Retinal cotton-wool spots.

5. Sjögren syndrome

 Look for

- Keratoconjunctivitis sicca.

6. Waldenström macroglobulinemia

 Look for

- Corneal crystals.
- Slow-flow retinopathy.
- Proptosis.

Sclerodactyly

Signs

- The fingers are tapered, flexed, shiny and creaseless with loss of finger pulps.

Systemic Associations

1. Scleroderma (Fig. 2.51)

 Look for

(*see* Raynaud phenomenon).

2. Dermatomyositis

 Signs

- The fingers may also show erythematous (colloidin) papules over the metacarpophalangeal or proximal interphalangeal joints (Gottron sign) (**Fig. 2.52**).

 Look for

(*see* Raynaud phenomenon).

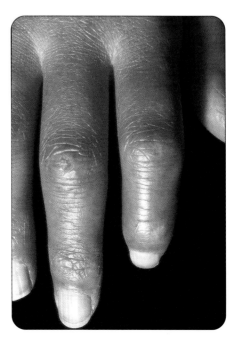

Fig. 2.52

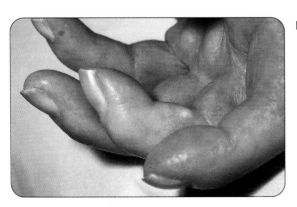

Fig. 2.51

Abnormal nails and nail beds

1. Pitting (Fig. 2.53)

 Look for

- Psoriatic arthritis.
- Eczema.

2. Onycholysis (Fig. 2.54).

Look for

- Psoriatic arthritis.

3. Nail dystrophy (Fig. 2.55)

Look for

- Epidermolysis bullosa.

4. White nails (leukonychia) (Fig. 2.56)

 Look for

- Liver disease.

5. Brown nail arcs (Fig. 2.57)

 Look for

- Renal disease.

6. Spoon-shaped nails (koilonychia) (Fig. 2.58)

 Look for

- Iron deficiency anemia.

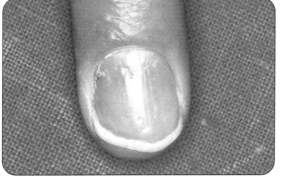

Fig. 2.53

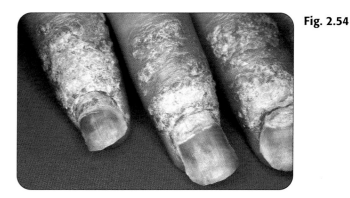

Fig. 2.54

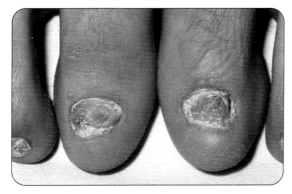

Fig. 2.55

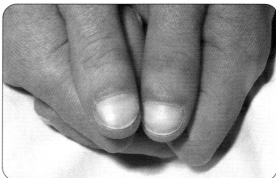

Fig. 2.56

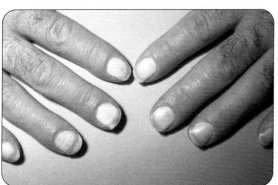

Fig. 2.57

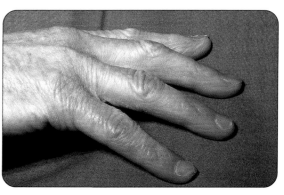

Fig. 2.58

7. Subungual splinter hemorrhages (Fig. 2.59)

 Look for

- Bacterial endocarditis.

8. Nail-fold infarcts (Fig. 2.60)

 Look for

- Rheumatoid arthritis.
- Systemic lupus erythematosus.
- Dermatomyositis.

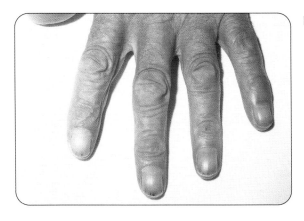

Fig. 2.59

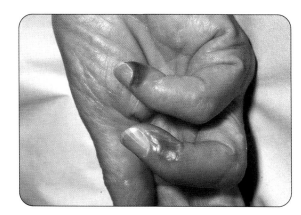

Fig. 2.60

THE HAIR

Alopecia and madarosis

Signs

- Alopecia is a decrease in number (**Fig. 2.61**) or a complete loss of hair (**Fig. 2.62**).

- Madarosis is a decrease in number or complete loss of lashes (**Fig. 2.63**).

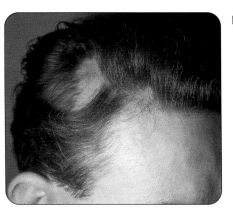

Fig. 2.61

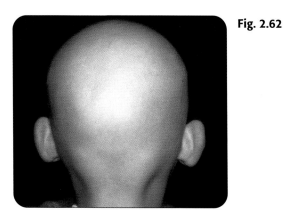

Fig. 2.62

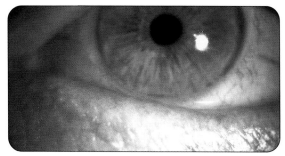

Fig. 2.63

Systemic Associations

1. Vogt–Koyanagi–Harada syndrome

 Look for

- Granulomatous anterior uveitis (Vogt–Koyanagi syndrome).
- Multifocal choroiditis and exudative retinal detachment (Harada disease).

2. Myxedema

 Look for

- Periorbital puffiness.
- Corneal arcus if the cholesterol level is raised.

3. Systemic lupus erythematosus

 Look for

- Keratoconjunctivitis sicca.
- Peripheral ulcerative keratitis.
- Retinal periarteritis.

4. Lepromatous leprosy

 Look for

- Anterior uveitis.
- Keratitis.

HIRSUTISM

Signs

- A male pattern of hair growth in a female (**Fig. 2.64**).

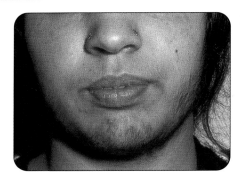

Fig. 2.64

Systemic Associations

1. Cushing syndrome

 Look for

- Steroid-related cataracts.
- Bitemporal hemianopia due to chiasmal compression by a pituitary basophil adenoma.

2. Acromegaly

 Look for

- Bitemporal hemianopia due to chiasmal compression by a pituitary acidophil adenoma.

3. Turner syndrome

 Look for

- Keratoconus.
- Blue sclera.

4. Porphyria cutanea tarda

 Look for

- Cicatrizing conjunctivitis.
- Scleritis.

Poliosis

Signs

- Poliosis is a premature, localized whitening of hair which may involve the lashes (**Fig. 2.65**) and eyebrows.
- It may be associated with vitiligo (*see* below).

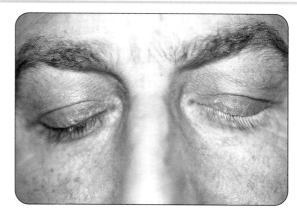

Fig. 2.65

Systemic Associations

1. Vogt–Koyanagi–Harada syndrome

 Look for

(*See* Alopecia and madarosis, p. 83.)

2. Waardenburg syndrome

 Look for

- Heterochromia iridis.
- Ocular albinism.

THE SKIN

Erythema nodosum

Signs

- Tender, erythematous nodules on the shins (**Fig. 2.66**) and occasionally on the thighs (**Fig. 2.67**) and forearms.

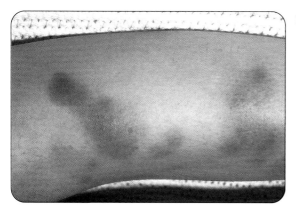

Fig. 2.66

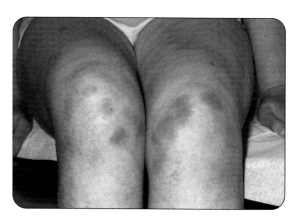

Fig. 2.67

Systemic Associations

1. Acute sarcoidosis (Löfgren syndrome)

 Look for

- Acute anterior uveitis.

2. Tuberculosis

 Look for

- Granulomatous anterior uveitis.
- Multifocal choroiditis.

3. Crohn disease

 Look for

- Acute anterior uveitis.
- Conjunctivitis.

4. Ulcerative colitis

 Look for

- Acute anterior uveitis.

5. Behçet disease

 Look for

- Acute anterior uveitis.
- Retinitis.
- Retinal periphlebitis and periarteritis.

6. Lepromatous leprosy

 Look for

- Anterior uveitis.
- Keratitis.

7. Coccidioidomycosis

 Look for

- Anterior uveitis.
- Multifocal choroiditis.

8. Cat-scratch fever

 Look for

- Parinaud oculoglandular syndrome.
- Intermediate uveitis.
- Neuroretinitis.

Vitiligo

Signs

- Well-defined, symmetrical areas of progressive depigmentation on the face (**Fig. 2.68**), neck (**Fig. 2.69**), groins, axillae, genitalia and the dorsum of the hands (**Fig. 2.70**).

- Hair in the involved area may become white (poliosis).

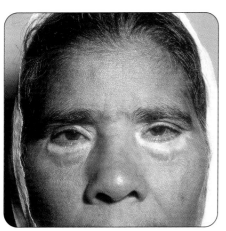
Fig. 2.68

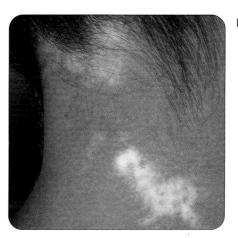
Fig. 2.69

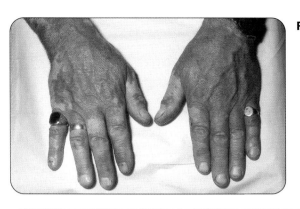

Fig. 2.70

Systemic Associations

1. Vogt–Koyanagi–Harada syndrome

 Look for

(*see* Alopecia and madarosis, p. 83.)

2. Other
- Myxedema.
- Thyrotoxicosis.
- Pernicious anemia.

Localized hypopigmented patches

Systemic Associations

1. Lepromatous leprosy

 Signs

- Numerous, hypopigmented macules (**Fig. 2.71**).

 Look for

- Anterior uveitis.
- Keratitis.

2. Tuberous sclerosis

 Signs

- Hypopigmented patches (ash leaf spots) on the trunk (**Fig. 2.72**), limbs and scalp (**Fig. 2.73**).

 Look for

- Retinal or optic disc astrocytomas which may be bilateral and multiple.

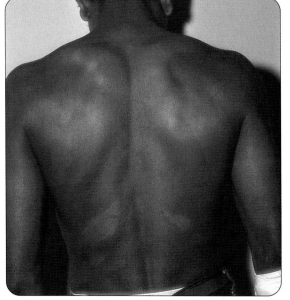

Fig. 2.71

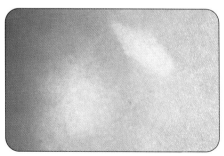

Fig. 2.72

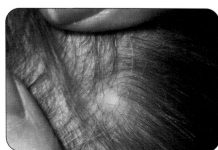

Fig. 2.73

Generalized hyperpigmentation

Systemic Associations

1. Hemochromatosis (Fig. 2.74)

 Look for

- Keratoconjunctivitis sicca.

2. Whipple disease

 Look for

- Intermediate uveitis.
- Retinal periphlebitis.

3. Cushing disease (Fig. 2.75)

 Look for

- Steroid-related cataracts.
- Bitemporal hemianopia due to chiasmal compression by a pituitary basophil adenoma.

4. Porphyria cutanea tarda

 Look for

- Cicatrizing conjunctivitis.
- Scleritis.

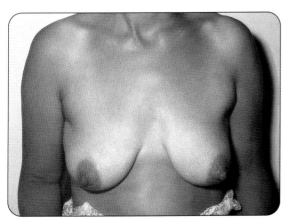

Fig. 2.74

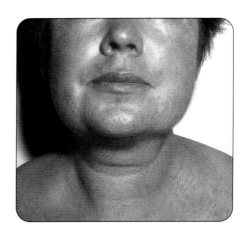

Fig. 2.75

Acanthosis nigricans

Signs

- Localized hyperpigmentation in the axillae and groins (**Fig. 2.76**).

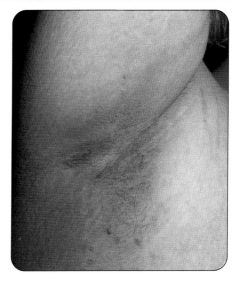

Fig. 2.76

Systemic Association

Carcinoma of stomach, breast or lung

 Look for

- Orbital or uveal metastases.
- Cancer-associated retinopathy.

Vesiculobullous dermatoses

Signs

- Blisters are visible accumulations of fluid. They can be subdivided into vesicles which are small and bullae which are larger than 1 cm.

Systemic Associations

1. Cicatricial pemphigoid

 Signs

- Mucosal involvement is universal.
- Skin blisters are chronic, usually sparse and heal by scarring (**Fig. 2.77**).

 Look for

- Cicatrizing conjunctivitis is very frequent.

2. Stevens–Johnson syndrome (erythema multiforme major)

 Signs

- Mucosal blisters are universal.

- Target skin lesions have a red center which is itself encircled by a peripheral red ring. They are most frequently develop on the palms and soles (**Fig. 2.78**).
- Skin blisters are usually transient but may be widespread and associated with hemorrhage and necrosis (**Fig. 2.79**).

 Look for

- Initially, transient membranous conjunctivitis is frequent.
- Later, cicatrizing conjunctivitis may develop in some cases.

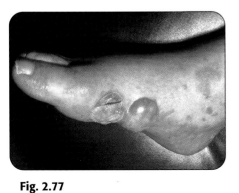

Fig. 2.77

Fig. 2.78

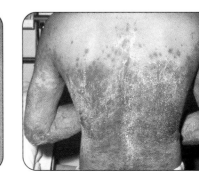

Fig. 2.79

3. Epidermolysis bullosa

 Signs

- Chronic skin blisters which develop following minor skin trauma (**Fig. 2.80**).
- Complications include partial fusion of the fingers and toes, and nail dystrophy.

 Look for

- Corneal erosions are frequent.
- Cicatrizing conjunctivitis is infrequent.

4. Pemphigus vulgaris

 Signs

- Mucosal involvement is frequent.
- Chronic widespread flaccid, thin-walled skin blisters that erode and leave large denuded areas (**Fig. 2.81**).

 Look for

- Conjunctivitis is infrequent and does not result in scarring.

5. Toxic epidermal necrolysis (Lyell disease, scalded skin syndrome)

 Signs

- Mucosal involvement is universal.
- Transient, painful, widespread skin blisters resembling scalded skin (**Fig. 2.82**).
- Subsequent epidermal loss can be precipitated by a lateral shearing force (Nikolsky sign).

 Look for

- Conjunctival involvement is similar to Stevens–Johnson syndrome but milder.

6. Pemphigoid

 Signs

- Mucosal involvement is frequent.
- Large, symmetrical, widespread skin blisters which are usually self-limiting an resolve without scarring (**Fig. 2.83**).

 Look for

- Cicatrizing conjunctivitis is infrequent.

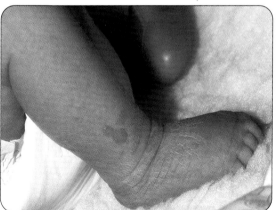

Fig. 2.80

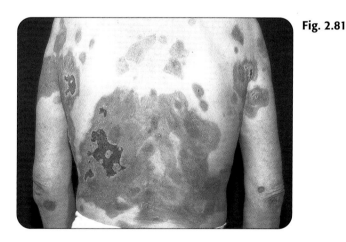

Fig. 2.81

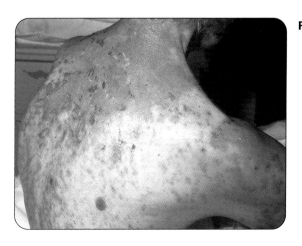

Fig. 2.82

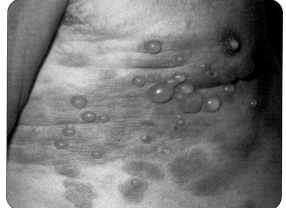

Fig. 2.83

7. Linear IgA disease (bullous dermatosis)

 Signs

- Mucosal involvement is very frequent.
- Tense skin blisters of varying size which are usually self-limiting (**Fig. 2.84**).

 Look for

- Cicatrizing conjunctivitis is very frequent.

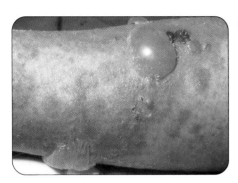

Fig. 2.84

8. Dermatitis herpetiformis

 Signs

- Groups of small itching blisters associated with urticaria which heal without scarring (**Fig. 2.85**).

 Look for

- Cicatrizing conjunctivitis is rare.

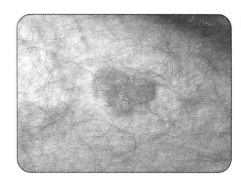

Fig. 2.85

Pyoderma gangrenosum

Signs

- Skin necrosis with irregular ulceration (**Fig. 2.86**).

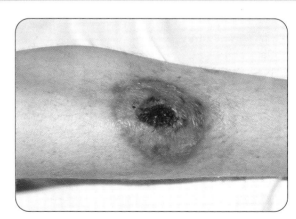

Fig. 2.86

Systemic Associations

1. Wegener granulomatosis

 Look for

- Peripheral ulcerative keratitis.
- Anterior scleritis.

2. Other

- Ulcerative colitis.
- Crohn disease.
- Rheumatoid arthritis.

Cutaneous bleeding

Signs

- Purpura is a small cutaneous extravasation of blood (**Fig. 2.87**).

- Echymosis or bruising is more extensive cutaneous bleeding (**Fig. 2.88**).

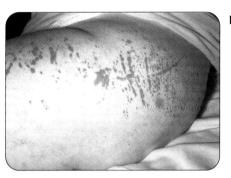

Fig. 2.87

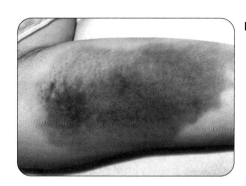

Fig. 2.88

Systemic Associations

1. Leukemias

 Look for

- Pseudo-hypopyon.
- Spontaneous hyphema.
- Retinal hemorrhages and cotton-wool spots.

2. Polycythemia rubra vera

 Look for

- Slow-flow retinopathy.
- Retinal vein occlusion.

3. Multiple myeloma

 Look for

- Corneal crystals.
- Slow-flow retinopathy.

4. Hermansky–Pudlak syndrome

 Look for

- Ocular albinism.

Thin hyperelastic skin

Signs

- Thin skin that can be easily stretched (**Fig. 2.89**).
- The skin bruises easily and heals slowly.

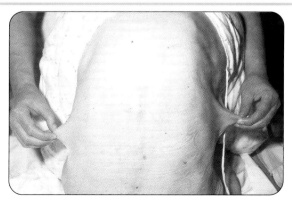

Fig. 2.89

Systemic Associations

1. Ehlers–Danlos syndrome type 6

 Look for

- High myopia and retinal detachment.
- Lens subluxation.
- Ocular fragility to trauma.
- Blue sclera and keratoconus.
- Angioid streaks.

2. Pseudoxanthoma elasticum

 Look for

- Blue sclera – only in dominant type 2.
- Angioid streaks – most severe in dominant type 1.

Vasculitis

Signs

- Palpable purpura which may progress to necrosis or bullae formation.

- Classically affects the lower parts of the legs (**Fig. 2.90**) but the arms (**Fig. 2.91**) and trunk can also be affected.

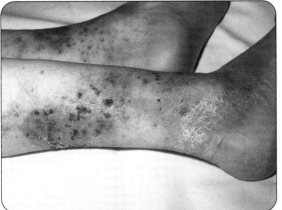

Fig. 2.90

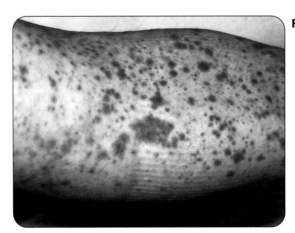

Fig. 2.91

Systemic Associations

1. Polyarteritis nodosa

 Look for

- Peripheral ulcerative keratitis.
- Anterior scleritis.
- Retinal periarteritis.

2. Rheumatoid arthritis

 Look for

- Keratoconjunctivitis sicca.
- Scleritis.
- Peripheral ulcerative keratitis.

3. Systemic lupus erythematosus

 Look for

- Keratoconjunctivitis sicca.
- Peripheral ulcerative keratitis.
- Retinal periarteritis.

4. Churg–Strauss syndrome

 Look for

- Scleritis.
- Retinal periarteritis.

Telangiectasia

Signs

- Dilated blood vessels which assume various shapes and blanch on pressure (**Fig. 2.92**).

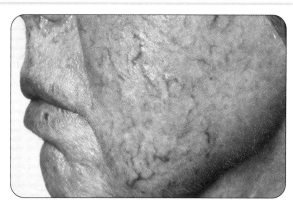

Fig. 2.92

Systemic Associations

1. Ataxia telangiectasia

 Look for

- Bulbar conjunctival telangiectasia.
- Ocular motility defects.

2. Fabry disease

 Look for

- Vortex keratopathy.

- Conjunctival telangiectasia.
- Congenital wedge-shaped cataracts.

3. Other
- Systemic lupus erythematosus.
- Systemic sclerosis.
- Dermatomyositis.

Livedo reticularis

Signs

- Persistent, patchy, reddish-blue mottling of the legs which tends to be worse in cold weather (**Fig. 2.93**).
- It is caused by spasm of cutaneous arterioles with secondary dilatation of capillaries and venules.

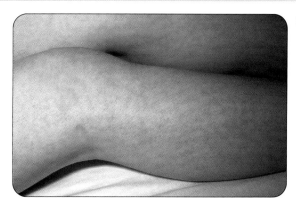

Fig. 2.93

Systemic Associations

1. Polyarteritis nodosa

 Look for

(*see* Vasculitis, p. 93)

2. Antiphospholipid antibody syndrome

 Look for

- Retinal cotton-wool spots and venous dilatation.
- Retinal arterial and venous occlusion.

Acquired ichthyosis

Signs

- Itchy dry and scaly skin which may be associated with hyperkeratosis (**Fig. 2.94**).

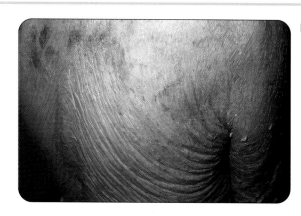

Fig. 2.94

Systemic Associations

1. Lymphoma

 Look for

- Mikulicz syndrome.
- Orbital and conjunctival involvement.
- Uveal infiltration.

2. Refsum disease

 Look for

- Pigmentary retinopathy.
- Prominent corneal nerves.
- Miosis.

Tumors

Systemic Associations

1. Xeroderma pigmentosum

 Look for

- Multiple malignant tumors (**Fig. 2.95**).

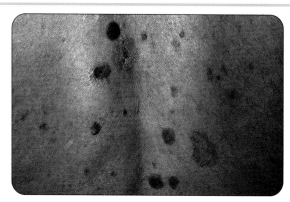

Fig. 2.95

2. Nevus of Ota

 Look for

- Melanoma (**Fig. 2.96**).

3. AIDS

 Look for

- Kaposi sarcoma (**Fig. 2.97**).
- Molluscum contagiosum (**Fig. 2.98**).

4. Neurofibromatosis–1

 Look for

- Plexiform neurofibromas (**Fig. 2.99**).
- Pedunculated neurofibromas (**Fig. 2.100**).

5. B-cell lymphoma

 Look for

- Firm, fleshy tumor (**Fig. 2.101**).

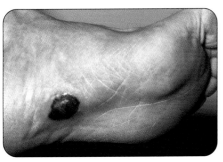
Fig. 2.96

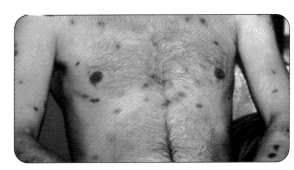
Fig. 2.97

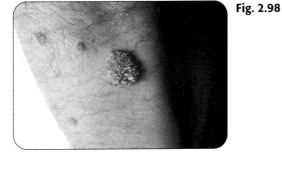
Fig. 2.98

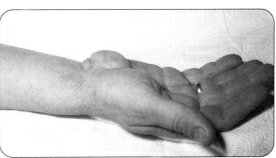
Fig. 2.99

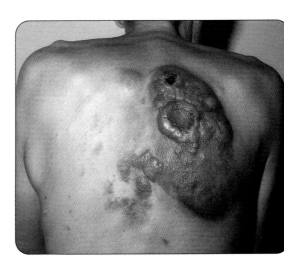
Fig. 2.100

Fig. 2.101

Granulomas

Signs

- Nodules or plaques which may be associated with secondary telangiectasia.

Systemic Associations

1. Sarcoidosis

 Signs

- Lupus pernio – indurated, soft, violaceous plaque with a predilection for the face, nose, cheeks and ears (**Fig. 2.102**).
- Papulonodular blue–red lesions on the limbs, shoulders and buttocks (**Fig. 2.103**).

 Look for

- Keratoconjunctivitis sicca.
- Anterior uveitis.
- Multifocal choroiditis.

2. Lepromatous leprosy

 Signs

- Plaques and nodules frequently on the nose and face (**Fig. 2.104**).

 Look for

- Anterior uveitis.
- Keratitis.

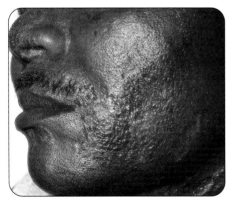

Fig. 2.102

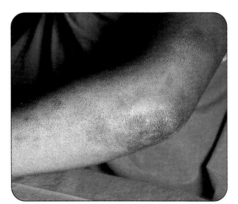

Fig. 2.103

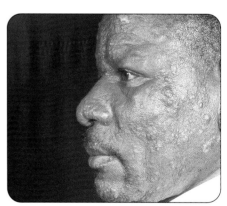

Fig. 2.104

3. Diabetes

 Signs

- Necrobiosis lipoidica – yellowish atrophic plaques with shiny atrophic centers on both shins (**Fig. 2.105**).
- Granuloma annulare – smooth plaques on the dorsum of the hands and feet, fingers, ankles and elbows (**Fig. 2.106**).

 Look for

- Retinopathy.
- Ocular motor nerve palsies.

4. Hyperlipoproteinemia

 Signs

- Xanthomata – firm, yellowish papules over the knees, elbows, heels and buttocks (**Fig. 2.107**).
- Tendon xanthomata occur in types II and III hyperlipidemia.

Look for

- Corneal arcus.
- Retinal vein occlusion.

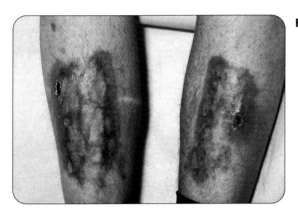

Fig. 2.105

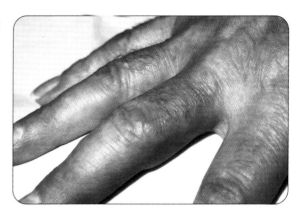

Fig. 2.106

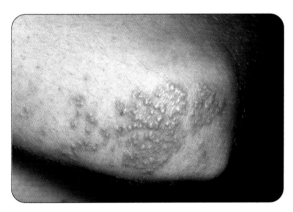

Fig. 2.107

THE JOINTS

Inflammatory arthritis

Signs

- Peripheral arthritis is characterized by swelling, stiffness and later deformity of peripheral joints.
- Sacroiliitis is characterized by pain and tenderness over the sacroiliac joints.
- Ankylosing spondylitis is characterized by stiffness and reduced mobility of the spine.

Systemic Association

1. Rheumatoid arthritis

 Signs

- Typically symmetrical arthritis of the hands (**Fig. 2.108**), ankles and knees.

 Look for

- Keratoconjunctivitis sicca.
- Scleritis.
- Peripheral ulcerative keratitis.

2. Juvenile idiopathic arthritis

 Signs

- Typically arthritis of the knees (**Fig. 2.109**), and less commonly the ankles and hands.

 Look for

- Chronic anterior uveitis.

3. Reiter syndrome

 Signs

- Typically arthritis of the lower limbs (**Fig. 2.110**).
- Frequently also spinal arthritis.

 Look for

- Conjunctivitis.
- Acute anterior uveitis.

4. Ankylosing spondylitis

 Signs

- Primarily spinal arthritis (**Fig. 2.111**).
- Also peripheral asymmetrical arthritis.

 Look for

- Acute anterior uveitis.

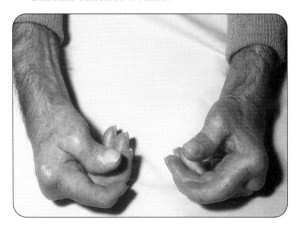
Fig. 2.108

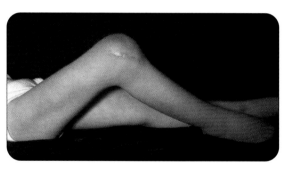
Fig. 2.109

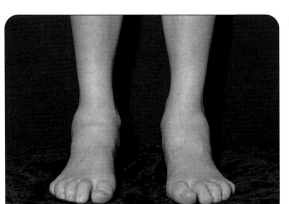
Fig. 2.110

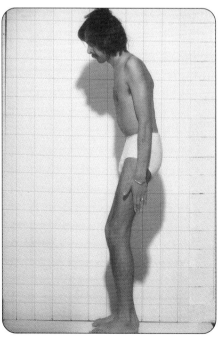
Fig. 2.111

5. Psoriatic arthritis

 Signs

- Typically asymmetrical arthritis of the knuckles and distal interphalangeal joints (**Fig. 2.112**).
- Frequently also spinal arthritis.

 Look for

- Acute anterior uveitis.
- Conjunctivitis.

6. Systemic lupus erythematosus

 Signs

- Arthritis may be similar to rheumatoid disease (**Fig. 2.113**).

 Look for

- Keratoconjunctivitis sicca.
- Peripheral ulcerative keratitis.
- Retinal periarteritis.

7. Behçet disease

 Signs

- Typically lower limb arthritis (**Fig. 2.114**).
- Occasionally spinal arthritis.

 Look for

- Acute anterior uveitis.
- Retinitis.
- Retinal periphlebitis.

8. Gout

 Signs

- Initially peripheral monoarthritis with erythema (**Fig. 2.115**).
- Later deforming arthritis with tophi (**Fig. 2.116**).

 Look for

- Corneal crystals.
- Band keratopathy.

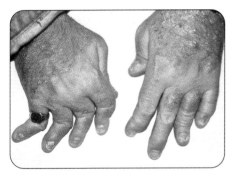

Fig. 2.112

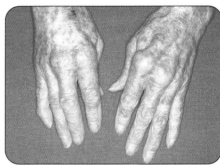
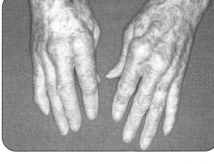

Fig. 2.113

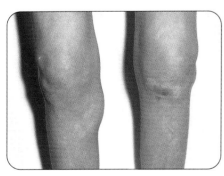

Fig. 2.114

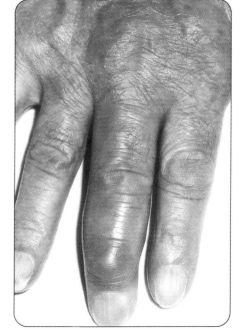

Fig. 2.115

Fig. 2.116

10. Ulcerative colitis

 Signs

- Mainly spinal arthritis.
- Also peripheral lower limb arthritis.

 Look for

- Acute anterior uveitis.

11. Crohn disease

 Signs

- Mainly spinal arthritis.
- Also peripheral lower limb arthritis.

 Look for

- Acute anterior uveitis.
- Conjunctivitis.

12. Whipple disease

 Signs

- Mainly migratory peripheral arthritis.
- Occasionally spinal arthritis.

 Look for

- Intermediate uveitis.
- Retinal periphlebitis.

Joint hypermobility

Systemic Associations

1. Marfan syndrome (Fig. 2.117).

 Look for

- Upward lens subluxation.
- Megalocornea and keratoconus.
- Retinal detachment.

2. Ehlers–Danlos syndrome (Fig. 2.118)

 Look for

- Lens subluxation.
- Angioid streaks.

3. Osteogenesis imperfecta type 1

 Look for

- Corneal arcus.
- Blue sclera.

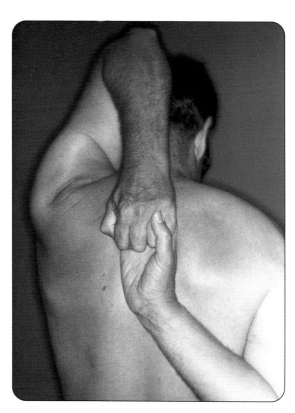

Fig. 2.118

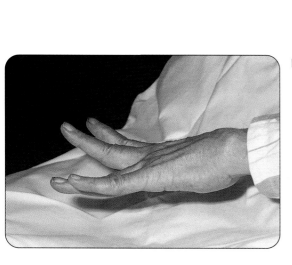

Fig. 2.117

Neuropathic (Charcot) arthropathy

Signs

- Loss of joint sensation resulting in osteoarthritis with new bone formation and instability (**Fig. 2.119**).

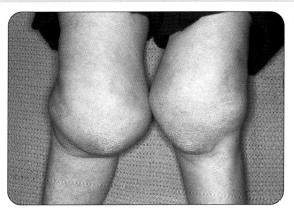

Fig. 2.119

SYSTEMIC ASSOCIATIONS

1. Diabetes

 Look for

- Retinopathy.
- Cataract.
- Ocular motor nerve palsies.

2. Syringomyelia

 Look for

- Horner syndrome.

3. Syphilis (tabes dorsalis)

 Look for

- Interstitial keratitis.
- Argyll Robertson pupils.

4. Charcot–Marie–Tooth disease

 Look for

- Optic atrophy.

THE LUNGS

Pulmonary infection and inflammation

Systemic Associations

1. Tuberculosis

 Signs

- Chronic fibrocaseous infection and cavitation (**Fig. 2.120**).

 Look for

- Granulomatous anterior uveitis.
- Multifocal choroiditis.

2. AIDS

 Signs

- *Pneumocystis carinii* pneumonia (**Fig. 2.121**).

 Look for

- Conjunctival and eyelid Kaposi sarcoma.
- HIV retinopathy.
- Cytomegalovirus retinitis.

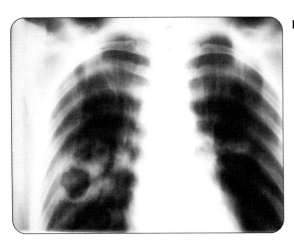

Fig. 2.120

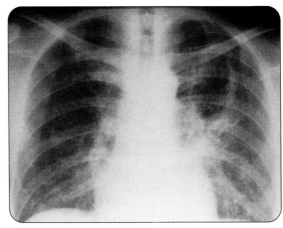

Fig. 2.121

3. Coccidioidomycosis

 Signs

- Chronic pulmonary infection.

 Look for

- Anterior uveitis.
- Multifocal choroiditis.

4. Histoplasmosis

 Signs

- Occasionally acute pulmonary infection with hilar adenopathy.

 Look for

- Multifocal choroiditis.
- Maculopathy associated with choroidal neovascularization.

5. Goodpasture syndrome

 Signs

- Hemoptysis, dyspnea and cough.

 Look for

- Retinal hemorrhages and cotton-wool spots.
- Exudative retinal detachment.

Pulmonary granulomatosis

Systemic Associations

1. Wegener granulomatosis

 Signs

- Pulmonary nodular lesions, infiltrates and cavities with fluid levels (**Fig. 2.122**).

 Look for

- Orbital involvement.
- Peripheral ulcerative keratitis.
- Scleritis.

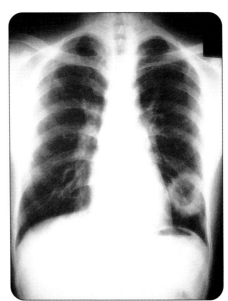

Fig. 2.122

2. Sarcoidosis

 Signs

- Hilar adenopathy, pulmonary parenchymal infiltrates and fibrosis (**Fig. 2.123**).

 Look for

- Keratoconjunctivitis sicca.
- Granulomatous anterior uveitis.
- Multifocal choroiditis.

3. Churg–Strauss syndrome

 Signs

- Hilar adenopathy, pulmonary infiltrates and nodules.

 Look for

- Scleritis.
- Retinal periarteritis.

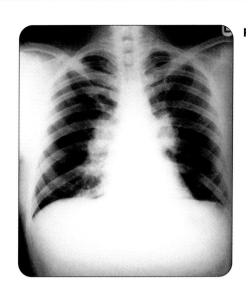

Fig. 2.123

THE CARDIOVASCULAR SYSTEM

Atheromatous vascular occlusion

Signs

- Coronary artery disease.
- Peripheral vascular disease and intermittent claudication.
- Ulceration of extremities (**Fig. 2.124**).
- Gangrene of extremities (**Fig. 2.125**).

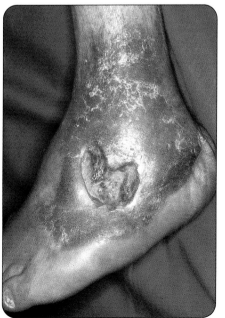

Fig. 2.124

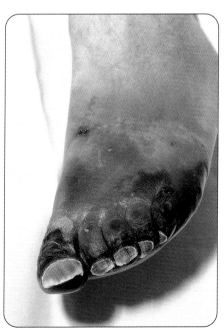

Fig. 2.125

SYSTEMIC ASSOCIATIONS

1. Diabetes

 Look for

- Retinopathy.
- Ocular motor palsies.

2. Hypertension

 Look for

- Retinopathy and retinal vein occlusion.
- Anterior ischemic optic neuropathy.
- Ocular motor nerve palsies.

3. Hyperlipoproteinemia

 Look for

- Eyelid xanthelasma.
- Cornea arcus.

- Retinal vein occlusion.
- Lipemia retinalis.

4. Pseudoxanthoma elasticum – dominant type 1

 Look for

- Angioid streaks.

5. Lecithin-cholesterol acetyltransferase deficiency

 Look for

- Corneal arcus-like clouding.

6. Cerebrotendinous xanthomatosis

 Look for

- Eyelid xanthelasma.
- Early-onset cataract.

Non-atheromatous vascular occlusion

Signs

- Peripheral arterial occlusion (**Fig. 2.126**).
- Superficial venous occlusion (**Fig. 2.127**).
- Deep venous occlusion of leg veins resulting in edema (**Fig. 2.128**).

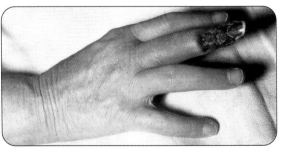

Fig. 2.126

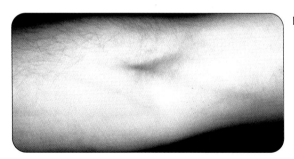

Fig. 2.127

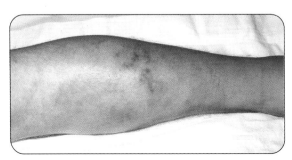

Fig. 2.128

- Occasionally occlusion of major internal veins which may result in the formation of superficial dilated by-pass channels (**Fig. 2.129**).

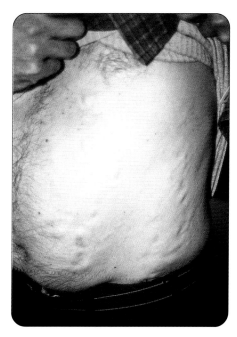

Fig. 2.129

SYSTEMIC ASSOCIATIONS

1. Homocystinuria

 Signs

- Thrombosis of any vessel at any age.

 Look for

- Inferior lens subluxation.
- Myopia and retinal detachment.

2. Antiphospholipid antibody syndrome

 Signs

- Arterial and venous thrombosis in young adults.

 Look for

- Retinal cotton-wool spots and venous dilatation.
- Retinal venous and arterial occlusion.
- Anterior ischemic optic neuropathy.

3. Behçet disease

 Signs

- Thrombosis of superficial veins, deep leg veins and occasionally of major internal veins.

4. Waldenström macroglobulinemia

 Signs

- Raynaud phenomenon, ulceration and gangrene of extremities.

 Look for

- Slow-flow retinopathy.
- Retinal cotton-wool spots.
- Corneal crystals.

Arteritis

Systemic Associations

1. Giant cell arteritis

 Signs

- Granulomatous arteritis of aorta and its major branches, especially the extracranial branches of the carotid, particularly the temporal (**Fig. 2.130**).

 Look for

- Anterior ischemic optic neuropathy.

2. Polyarteritis nodosa

 Signs

- Necrotizing inflammation of medium and small arteries.

 Look for

- Scleritis.
- Peripheral ulcerative keratitis.
- Retinal periarteritis.

3. Takayasu disease

 Signs

- Granulomatous inflammation of the aorta and its major branches.

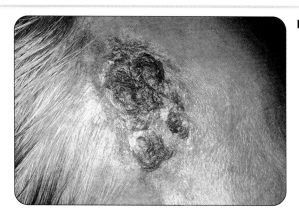

Fig. 2.130

 Look for

- Slow-flow retinopathy.
- Ocular ischemic syndrome.

4. Kawasaki disease

 Signs

- Childhood arteritis principally affecting the coronary arteries.

 Look for

- Acute conjunctivitis.
- Retinal periarteritis.

Heart valve disease

Systemic Associations

1. Bacterial endocarditis

 Signs

- Previously diseased or prosthetic valves (**Fig. 2.131**).

 Look for

- Retinal Roth spots.
- Retinal artery occlusion.

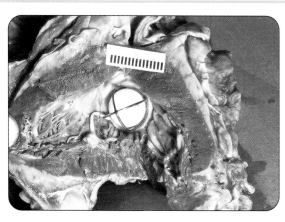

Fig. 2.131

2. Ankylosing spondylitis

 Signs

- Aortic incompetence.

 Look for

- Acute anterior uveitis.

3. Reiter syndrome

 Signs

- Aortic incompetence.

 Look for

- Acute conjunctivitis.
- Acute anterior uveitis.

4. Ehlers–Danlos syndrome

 Signs

- Mitral valve disease.

 Look for

- Lens subluxation.
- Angioid streaks.

5. Marfan syndrome

 Signs

- Aortic incompetence and mitral valve disease.

 Look for

- Upward lens subluxation.
- Megalocornea and keratoconus.
- Retinal detachment.

6. Down syndrome

 Signs

- Variable valve lesions which may be multiple.

 Look for

- Brushfield iris spots.
- Keratoconus.
- Cataract.

7. Pseudoxanthoma elasticum-dominant type 1

 Signs

- Mitral valve disease.

 Look for

- Angioid streaks.

8. Relapsing polychondritis

 Signs

- Variable valve disease and aortic artery involvement.

 Look for

- Scleritis.
- Peripheral ulcerative keratitis.

9. Osteogenesis imperfecta type 1

 Signs

- Aortic incompetence and mitral valve disease.

 Look for

- Blue sclera.
- Corneal arcus.

THE GASTROINTESTINAL TRACT

Inflammatory bowel disease

Signs

- Weight loss (**Fig. 2.132**).
- Diarrhea which may be bloody.
- Associations include arthritis, sclerosing cholangitis and pyoderma gangrenosum.

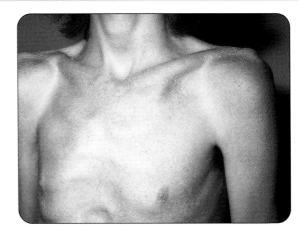

Fig. 2.132

Systemic Associations

1. Ulcerative colitis

 Look for

- Acute anterior uveitis.

2. Crohn disease

 Look for

- Acute anterior uveitis.
- Conjunctivitis.

3. Whipple disease

 Look for

- Intermediate uveitis.
- Retinal periphlebitis.

Intestinal malabsorption

Signs

- Anorexia, weight loss and lethargy.
- Abdominal discomfort and distension.
- Diarrhea and steatorrhea.
- Nutritional deficiencies.

Systemic Associations

1. Bassen–Kornzweig syndrome

 Look for

- Ptosis and progressive external ophthalmoplegia.
- Pigmentary retinopathy.

2. Cerebrotendinous xanthomatosis

 Look for

- Eyelid xanthelasma.
- Early-onset cataracts.

Intestinal adenomatous polyposis and carcinoma

Systemic Associations

1. Gardner syndrome

 Look for

- Atypical congenital hypertrophy of the retinal pigment epithelium.

2. Turcot syndrome

 Look for

- Atypical congenital hypertrophy of the retinal pigment epithelium.

Esophageal dysmobility and dysphagia

Systemic Associations

1. Systemic sclerosis

 Look for

- Keratoconjunctivitis sicca.
- Retinal cotton-wool spots

2. Myasthenia gravis

 Look for

- Ptosis.
- Diplopia.

3. Polymyositis

 Look for

- Keratoconjunctivitis sicca.
- Scleritis.
- Retinal cotton-wool spots.

4. Sjögren syndrome

 Look for

- Keratoconjunctivitis sicca.

5. Oculopharyngeal dystrophy

 Look for

- Ptosis.
- Progressive external ophthalmoplegia.

Liver disease

Signs

- Jaundice (**Fig. 2.133**).
- Palmar erythema (**Fig. 2.134**).
- Spider nevi (**Fig. 2.135**).
- Hepatomegaly and ascites (**Fig. 2.136**).
- Gynacomastia (**Fig. 2.137**).
- Finger clubbing and white nails.
- Encephalopathy.
- Bleeding diathesis.

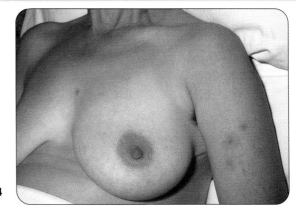

Fig. 2.133

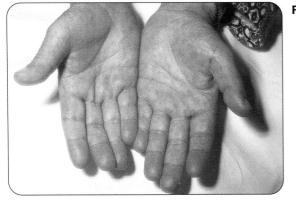

Fig. 2.134

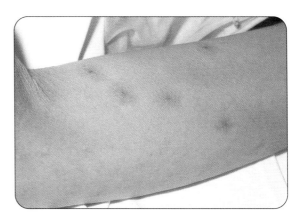

Fig. 2.135

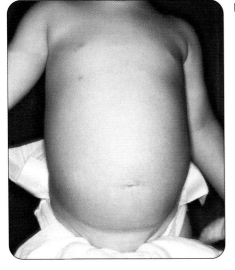

Fig. 2.136

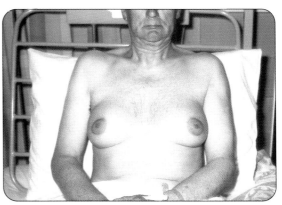

Fig. 2.137

SYSTEMIC ASSOCIATIONS

1. Wilson disease

 Look for

- Kayser–Fleischer ring.
- Sunflower cataract.

2. Primary biliary cirrhosis

 Look for

- Keratoconjunctivitis sicca.

THE KIDNEYS

Nephritis

Signs

- Proteinuria, hematuria, dysuria and oliguria.
- Pitting edema of the face (**Fig. 2.138**), abdomen and ankles occurs in the nephrotic syndrome.

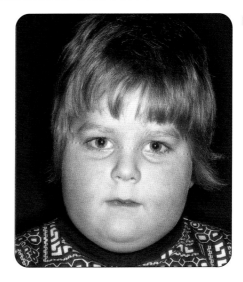

Fig. 2.138

Systemic Associations

1. Tubulointerstitial nephritis

 Look for

- Anterior uveitis.

2. IgA nephropathy

 Look for

- Anterior uveitis.
- Scleritis

3. Hemorrhagic nephritis in Alport syndrome

 Look for

- Anterior lenticonus and flecked retinopathy.

4. Membranoproliferative glomerulonephritis type 2

 Look for

- Bilateral, diffuse, yellow, drusen-like deposits at the posterior poles.

Secondary renal disease

Systemic Associations

1. Diabetes

 Look for

- Retinopathy.
- Ocular motor nerve palsies.

2. Hypertension

 Look for

- Retinopathy and retinal vein occlusion.
- Anterior ischemic optic neuropathy.
- Ocular motor nerve palsies.

3. Systemic lupus erythematosus

 Look for

- Keratoconjunctivitis sicca.
- Peripheral ulcerative keratitis.
- Retinal periarteritis.

4. Wegener granulomatosis

 Look for

- Orbital involvement.
- Scleritis.
- Peripheral ulcerative keratitis.

5. Goodpasture syndrome

 Look for

- Retinal cotton-wool spots and hemorrhages.
- Exudative retinal detachment.

6. Cystinosis – infantile neuropathic and intermediate adolescent

 Look for

- Corneal crystals.
- Pigmentary retinopathy.

7. Other
- Oxalosis.
- Lecithin-cholesterol acetyltransferase deficiency.
- Fabry disease.
- Antiphospholipid antibody syndrome.
- Churg–Strauss syndrome.

THE GENITALIA

Ulceration

Systemic Associations

1. Behçet disease

 Signs

- Recurrent ulceration of the penis or scrotum (**Fig. 2.139**) in males and of the labia and vagina in females.

 Look for

- Acute anterior uveitis.
- Retinitis.
- Retinal periphlebitis and periarteritis.

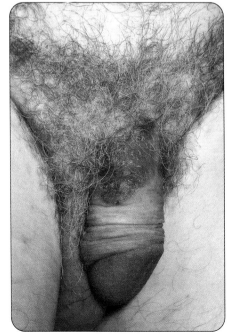

Fig. 2.139

2. Stevens–Johnson syndrome

 Signs

- Bullae and erosions of the glans penis (**Fig. 2.140**).

 Look for

- Initially transient membranous conjunctivitis.
- Later conjunctival cicatrization.

3. Reiter disease

 Signs

- Painless erythematous erosion of the gland penis (circinate balanitis) (**Fig. 2.141**).

 Look for

- Acute conjunctivitis.
- Acute anterior uveitis.

4. Acquired syphilis

 Signs

- Painless genital ulcer (chancre) and regional lymphadenopathy.

 Look for

- Anterior uveitis.

5. Chancroid

 Signs

- Genital ulceration and regional lymphadenopathy.

 Look for

- Parinaud oculoglandular syndrome.

6. Lymphogranuloma venereum

 Signs

- Painless genital ulceration and painful regional lymphadenopathy.

 Look for

- Parinaud oculoglandular syndrome.
- Interstitial keratitis.

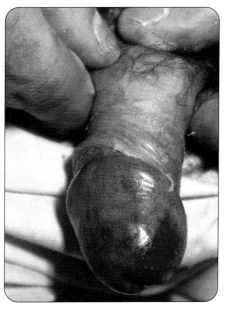

Fig. 2.140

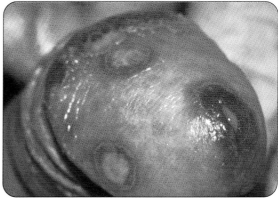

Fig. 2.141

Urethritis

Signs

- Urethral discharge and dysuria.

Systemic Associations

1. Chlamydial infection

 Look for

- Follicular conjunctivitis.
- Superior corneal micropannus.

2. Gonorrhea

 Look for

- Acute purulent conjunctivitis.

3. Reiter syndrome

 Look for

(*see* Ulceration).

THE NERVOUS SYSTEM

Peripheral neuropathy

Definitions and Signs

a. *Mononeuropthy* involves an isolated peripheral nerve such as the ulnar (**Fig. 2.142**).

b. *Multifocal neuropathy* (mononeuritis multiplex) involves multiple isolated nerves.

c. *Polyneuropathy* is characterized by diffuse or bilateral symmetrical involvement.

d. *Sensory neuropathy* is characterized by loss of sensation and in advanced cases it may result in perforating ulcers of the feet located at maximal pressure points (**Fig. 2.143**) and neuropathic (Charcot) joint degeneration.

e. *Motor neuropathy* is characterized by weakness, wasting and decreased tendon reflexes.

f. *Autonomic neuropathy* is characterized by disturbances of sphincter function and other features of autonomic dysfunction.

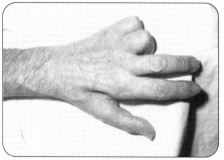
Fig. 2.142

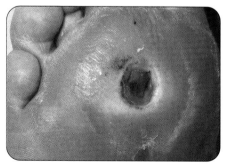
Fig. 2.143

Systemic Associations

1. Diabetes

 Signs

- Most frequently sensory polyneuropathy involving the feet.

 Look for

- Retinopathy.
- Ocular motor nerve palsies.

2. Sarcoidosis

 Signs

- Most frequently multifocal neuropathy with a predilection for the facial nerve (**Fig. 2.144**).

 Look for

- Keratoconjunctivitis sicca.
- Anterior uveitis.
- Multifocal choroiditis.

3. Polyarteritis nodosa

 Signs

- Multifocal neuropathy.

 Look for

- Scleritis.
- Peripheral ulcerative keratitis.

4. Wegener granulomatosis

 Signs

- Multifocal neuropathy.

 Look for

- Orbital involvement.
- Scleritis.
- Peripheral ulcerative keratitis.

5. Pernicious anemia

 Signs

- Most frequently sensory polyneuropathy principally affecting the lower parts of the legs.

 Look for

- Optic neuropathy.

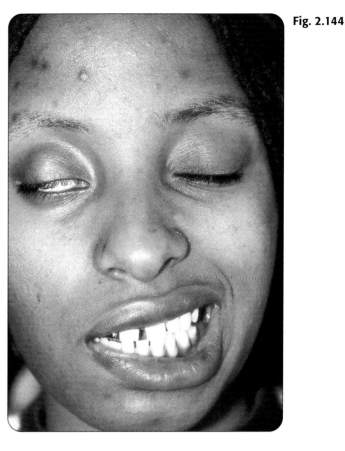

Fig. 2.144

6. Rheumatoid arthritis

 Signs

- Multifocal neuropathy.

 Look for

- Keratoconjunctivitis sicca.
- Scleritis.
- Peripheral ulcerative keratitis.

7. Primary amyloidosis

 Signs

- Initially sensory and later motor polyneuropathy.

 Look for

- Vitreous opacities.
- Prominent corneal nerves.
- Light–near dissociation of pupillary reaction.

4. von Hi

Signs

- Hemangi
  Fig. 2.14
  fossa hen

Look

- Retinal c
  and bilat

5. Neurof

Signs

- Optic ne
  is a sagi
  thalamu:

Look

- Lisch no
- Eyelid pl
- Optic ne

6. Neurof

Signs

- Bilateral

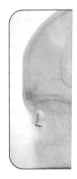

1. Paget

Loo

- Optic a
- Proptos
- Angioid

8. Lepromatous leprosy

Signs

- Sensory neuropathy resulting in shortening of digits (**Fig. 2.145**).

Look for

- Anterior uveitis.
- Keratitis

9. Charcot–Marie–Tooth disease

Signs

- Motor and sensory neuropathy initially involving the lower legs and later the small muscles of the hand (**Fig. 2.146**).

Look for

- Optic atrophy.

10. Refsum disease

Signs

- Mixed motor and sensory polyneuropathy.

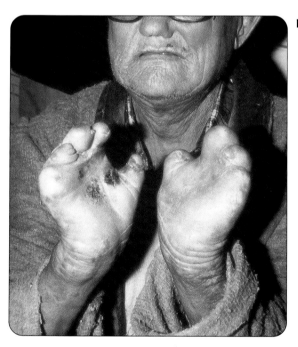
Fig. 2.145

Look for

- Pigmentary retinopathy.
- Prominent corneal nerves.
- Miotic pupils.

11. Lyme disease

Signs

- Initially cranial and later predominantly peripheral neuropathy.

Look for

- Conjunctivitis.
- Intermediate uveitis.

12. Churg–Strauss disease

Signs

- Multifocal neuropathy.

Look for

- Scleritis.
- Retinal periarteritis.

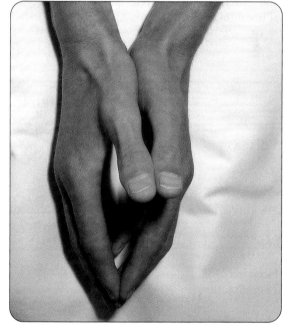
Fig. 2.146

ACROMEGALY

• This is an uncommon condition caused by a growth hormone secreting pituitary acidophil adenoma (**Fig. 3.1**).
• Ocular manifestations are frequent and serious.

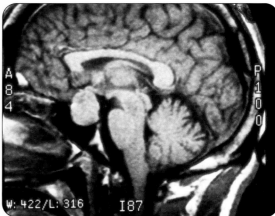

Fig. 3.1

Systemic features

 Presentation

• Frequently in the fourth and fifth decades with a very insidious onset.

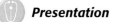 *Signs*

• Cutaneous hyperhidrosis, greasiness, acne, and in females, hirsutism.
• Facial coarseness with thick lips, exaggerated nasolabial folds and enlargement of the lower jaw with malocclusion (**Fig. 3.2**).

• Enlargement of the head, hands and feet (**Fig. 3.3**).
• Enlargement of tongue (macroglossia) and organomegaly.

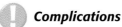 *Complications*

• Osteoarthritis and carpal tunnel syndrome.
• Cardiomyopathy, respiratory disease and hypertension.
• Diabetes and gonadal dysfunction.
• Neuropathy.

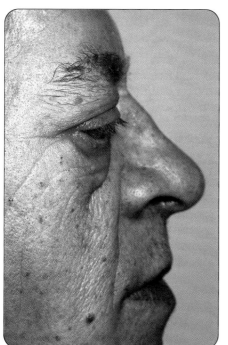

Fig. 3.2

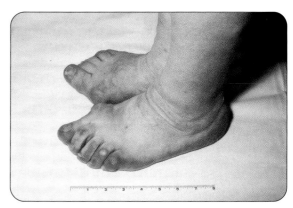

Fig. 3.3

Eye signs

- *Bitemoporal hemianopia due to chiasmal compression by the tumor* (**Fig. 3.4**).
- Optic atrophy.
- Diplopia.
- Angioid streaks.

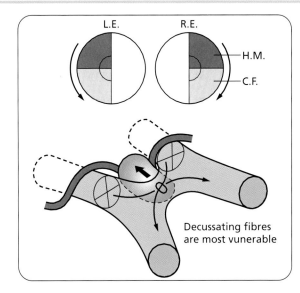

Fig. 3.4

ACQUIRED IMMUNE DEFICIENCY SYNDROME (AIDS)

- This is a common condition caused by the human immunodeficiency virus (HIV) which is predominantly transmitted by sexual intercourse and occasionally by contaminated blood or syringes.

- Ocular manifestations are frequent and serious.

Systemic features

Presentation

- May be asymptomatic or as a glandular fever-like illness which is then followed by persistent lymphadenopathy.

Signs

Opportunistic infections

a. *Protozoan – Pneumocystis carinii* pneumonia or disseminated disease, and toxoplasmosis.

b. *Viral* – cytomegalovirus pneumonitis and colitis, and persistent invasive herpes simplex lesions.
c. *Fungal* – cryptococcosis and esophageal candidiasis.
d. *Bacterial* – atypical mycobacterial and extrapulmonary tuberculosis.

Tumors
- Kaposi sarcoma, molluscum contagiosum and non-Hodgkin lymphoma.

Eye signs

Eyelids
- Kaposi sarcoma (**Fig. 3.5**).
- Multiple molluscum lesions (**Fig. 3.6**).
- Severe herpes zoster ophthalmicus (**Fig. 3.7**).

Orbit
- Cellulitis usually from contiguous sinus infection (**Fig. 3.8**).
- B-cell lymphoma.

Anterior segment
- Kaposi sarcoma of the conjunctiva (**Fig. 3.9**).
- Keratoconjunctivitis sicca.
- Conjunctival microangiopathy.
- Chronic microsporidial keratoconjunctivitis.
- Herpes simplex keratitis (**Fig. 3.10**).
- Anterior uveitis.

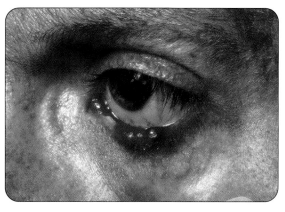

Fig. 3.5

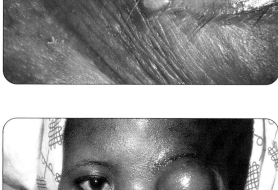

Fig. 3.6

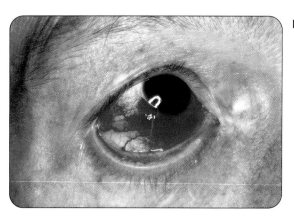

Fig. 3.7

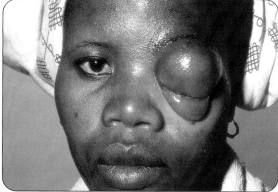

Fig. 3.8

Fig. 3.9

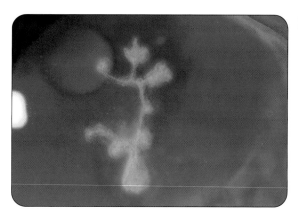

Fig. 3.10

Posterior segment
- HIV retinopathy characterized by cotton-wool spots.
- Cytomegalovirus retinitis (**Fig. 3.11**).
- Progressive outer retinal necrosis.
- *Pneumocystis carinii* choroiditis.
- Toxoplasma retinitis which may be atypical.
- Cryptococcal choroiditis.
- B-cell intraocular lymphoma.

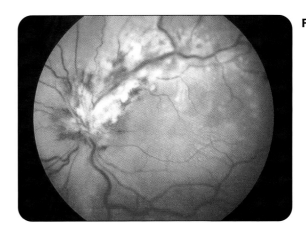

Fig. 3.11

ALKAPTONURIA

- This is a rare inborn error of metabolism caused by a defect in homogentistic acid oxidase with subsequent accumulation of homogentistic acid in tissues.
- Inheritance is autosomal recessive.
- Ocular manifestations are frequent but innocuous.

Systemic features

 Presentation

- In infancy with dark discoloration of urine.

 Signs

- *Grayish pigmentation of nasal cartilage and ear lobes.*
- Dark sweat stains of clothes.

Complications

- Premature disc degeneration of the spine.
- Arthropathy which may resemble rheumatoid arthritis.

Eye signs

- Greyish pigmentation of the interpalpebral sclera and tendons of the horizontal recti.
- 'Oil-droplet' corneal pigmentation just inside the limbus.

ALPORT SYNDROME

- This is a rare renal disorder caused by abnormal glomerular basement-membrane.
- Inheritance is X-linked dominant.
- Ocular manifestations are frequent but innocuous.

Systemic features

 Presentation

- Hematuria during the first year of life.

 Signs

- Progressive hemorrhagic nephritis.
- Bilateral sensorineural deafness.

 Complications

- Nephrotic syndrome and eventual renal failure.

Eye signs

- Anterior lenticonus.
- Flecked retinopathy (**Fig. 3.12**).

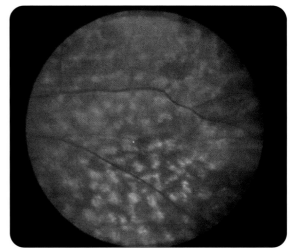

Fig. 3.12

AMYLOIDOSIS – HEREDITARY SYSTEMIC

- This is a rare metabolic disorder which is characterized by extracellular deposition of abnormal protein fibrils.

- Inheritance is autosomal dominant.
- Ocular manifestations are uncommon.

Systemic features

 Presentation

- At any time between the second and seventh decades with initially sensory, and later motor and autonomic polyneuropathy.

 Signs

- Variable visceral involvement of the heart, kidneys, thyroid and adrenals.

Eye signs

- *Vitreous opacities.*
- Prominent corneal nerves.
- Light–near dissociation of pupillary reactions.

ANEMIAS

- These are a common group of conditions characterized by either a decrease in the number of circulating red blood cells, a decrease in the amount of hemoglobin in each cell, or both.
- Except for sickle-cell anemia, ocular manifestations are rare and usually innocuous.

Systemic features

 Presentation

- At any age with fatigue and weakness.

 Signs

- Pallor of the skin and mucous membranes (**Fig. 3.13**) is common to all anemias.
- a. *Iron deficiency anemia*
- Koilonychia and brittle nails.
- Atrophic glossitis.
- Angular stomatitis (**Fig. 3.14**).

b. *Pernicious anemia*
- Vitiligo (**Fig. 3.15**).
- Premature graying of hair.
- Sensory polyneuropathy principally affecting the lower parts of the legs.
c. *Sickle–cell anemia*
- Splenomegaly.
d. *Aplastic anemia*
- Purpura.

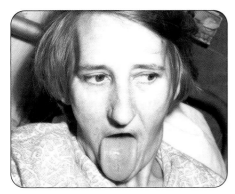

Fig. 3.13

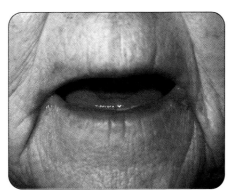

Fig. 3.14

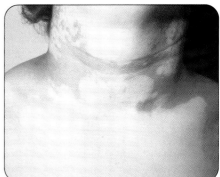

Fig. 3.15

Eye signs

- *Proliferative retinopathy in sickle-cell anemia.*
- *Optic neuropathy in pernicious anemia.*
- Retinal flame-shaped hemorrhages, cotton-wool spots, Roth spots and venous tortuosity in other anemias.

ANKYLOSING SPONDYLITIS

- This is a common, idiopathic, inflammatory arthropathy which primarily involves the sacro-iliac joints and axial skeleton (spondarthropathy) (**Fig. 3.16**).
- It typically affects males who carry HLA-B27.
- Ocular manifestations are frequent and potentially serious.

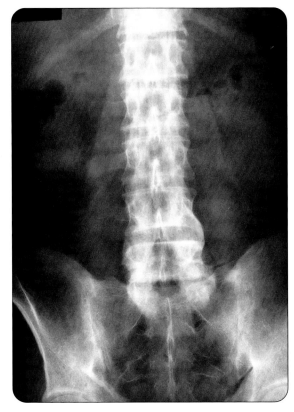

Fig. 3.16

Systemic features

 Presentation

- Prior to the age of 40 years with insidious onset of pain and stiffness in the low back or buttocks.

 Signs

- Progressive limitation of spinal movements.
- Peripheral asymmetrical polyarthritis.
- Enthesopathy of the plantar fascia and Achilles tendon.

 Associations

- Inflammatory bowel disease.
- Apical pulmonary fibrosis.
- Aortitis with secondary aortic incompetence.
- Cardiac conduction defects (atrioventricular block).

Eye signs

- *Acute recurrent anterior uveitis.*

- Conjunctivitis.

ANTIPHOSPHOLIPID ANTIBODY SYNDROME – PRIMARY

- This is a rare but potentially life-threatening prethrombotic autoimmune disease.
- It occurs in patients who do not have systemic lupus erythematosus but are positive for antiphospholipid antibody.
- Ocular manifestations are infrequent but serious.

Systemic features

 Presentation

- Arterial and venous thromboses in young adults.
- Recurrent spontaneous abortions.

 Signs

- Purpura.

- Venous thromboembolism in unusual sites such as cerebral venous sinuses and hepatic veins.
- Heart valve abnormalities.
- Renal disease.
- Livedo reticularis.

Eye signs

- *Retinal cotton-wool spots and venous dilation.*
- *Retinal venous occlusion* (**Fig. 3.17**).
- *Retinal arterial occlusion.*
- Anterior ischemic optic neuropathy.
- Transient visual loss.
- Conjunctival telangiectasia.

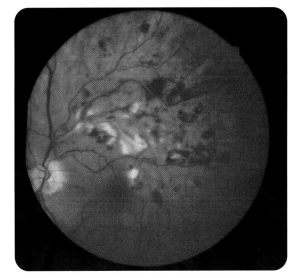

Fig. 3.17

ATAXIA TELANGIECTASIA (LOUIS–BAR SYNDROME)

- This is a rare neurocutaneous syndrome.
- Inheritance is autosomal recessive.

- Ocular manifestations are frequent but usually innocuous.

135

Systemic features

 Presentation

- During early childhood with ataxia, parkinsonian features and choreoathetosis.

 Signs

- Skin telangiectasia involving the pinnae, face and limb flexures.

 Associations

- Lymphopenia, immune deficit and hematopoietic malignancy.

Eye signs

- *Bulbar conjunctival telangiectasia.*

- Ocular motility disorders (supranuclear palsy, nystagmus, and oculomotor apraxia.)

ATOPIC ECZEMA

- This is a common, idiopathic, frequently familial skin condition which may be associated with asthma and hay fever.

- Ocular manifestations are frequent and may be persistent.

Systemic features

 Presentation

- Usually 3 months after birth but can be at any time with intense pruritis.

 Signs

- In babies, dry, erythematous itchy papules form on the face (**Fig. 3.18**).
- Later there is more generalized involvement.

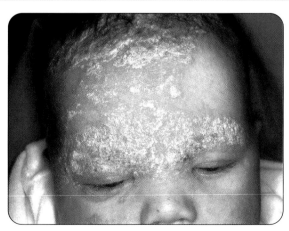

Fig. 3.18

! Complications

- Secondary infection may exacerbate eczema (**Fig. 3.19**).
- Lichenification due to constant rubbing and scratching.
- Disseminated herpes simplex infection (eczema herpeticum).

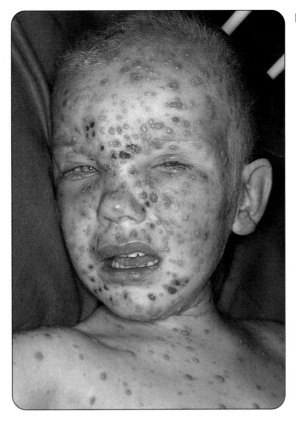

Fig. 3.19

Eye signs

- *Staphylococcal blepharitis and madarosis* (**Fig. 3.20**).
- *Chronic atopic keratoconjunctivitis* (**Fig. 3.21**).
- Anterior shield-like cataract.
- Keratoconus.
- Retinal detachment.

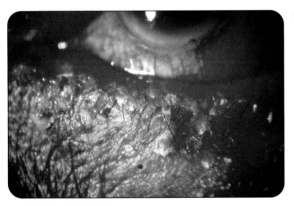

Fig. 3.20

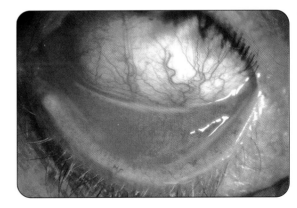

Fig. 3.21

BACTERIAL ENDOCARDITIS

- This is an uncommon disease characterized by bacterial inflammation of the lining of the heart chambers, heart valves and greater vessels.

- Patients with pre-existing cardiac abnormalities such as damaged or prosthetic valves, and congenital defects are at increased risk.
- Ocular manifestations are infrequent but serious.

Systemic features

 Presentation

- At any age with fever, night sweats, arthralgia and fatigue.

 Signs

- Heart murmurs.
- Finger clubbing.
- Splenomegaly.

- Petechial hemorrhages in the skin and under the nails (splinter hemorrhages).
- Osler's nodes which are purple, painful, tender lesions on the fingers and toes.
- Janeway lesions which are non-tender, erythematous maculae or nodules on the palms and soles.

 Complications

- Renal and neurological diseases.

Eye signs

- *Roth spots.*
- Endogenous endophthalmitis with hypopyon (**Fig. 3.22**).

- Subconjunctival hemorrhages (**Fig. 3.23**).
- Retinal artery occlusion.

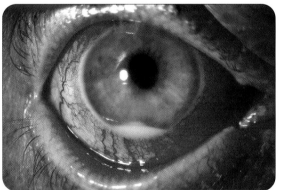

Fig. 3.22

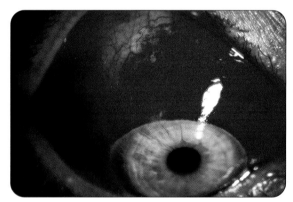

Fig. 3.23

BASSEN–KORNZWEIG SYNDROME

- This is a rare disease characterized by deficiency in beta-lipoprotein resulting in malabsorption and secondary vitamin A deficiency.

- Inheritance is autosomal recessive.
- Ocular manifestations are frequent and serious.

Systemic features

 Presentation

- In adolescence with steatorrhea and ataxia.

 Signs

- Spinocerebellar ataxia.
- Acanthocytosis in the peripheral blood.

Eye signs

- *Pigmentary retinopathy* (**Fig. 3.24**).
- *Ptosis and progressive external ophthalmoplegia.*

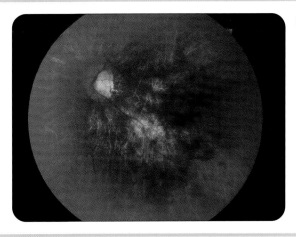

Fig. 3.24

BEHÇET DISEASE

- This is an uncommon, idiopathic, multisystem disease which typically affects young men from the eastern Mediterranean region and Japan.
- It is associated with an increased incidence of HLA-B51.
- Ocular manifestations are frequent and serious.

Systemic features

 Presentation

- In the third and fourth decades with localized lesions such as aphthous ulceration.

 Major diagnostic criteria

a. *Recurrent oral aphthous stomatitis.*
b. *Skin lesions*

- Erythema nodosum-like (**Fig. 3.25**).
- Acneiform (**Fig. 3.26**).
- Vasculitis.
- Hypersensitivity (dermatographism) (**Fig. 3.27**).
c. *Recurrent genital ulceration*
- Of the penis (**Fig. 3.28**) and scrotum in males.
- Of the labia and vagina in females.
d. *Uveitis.*

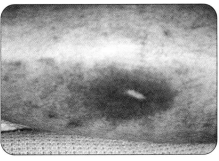

Fig. 3.25

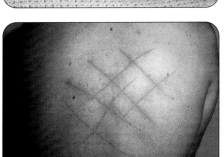

Fig. 3.27

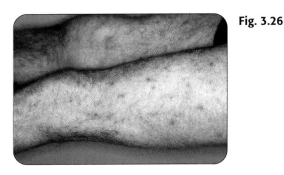

Fig. 3.26

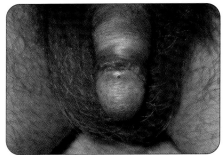

Fig. 3.28

Minor diagnostic criteria

a. *Arthritis* of the knees and ankles, and occasionally sacroiliitis.
b. *Epididymitis*.
c. *Intestinal ulceration*.
d. *Vascular lesions*.

- Obliterative thrombophlebitis.
- Arterial occlusion.
- Aneurysm formation.
e. *Central nervous system lesions*.
- Brainstem syndromes.
- Meningoencephalitis.

Eye signs

- *Acute anterior uveitis, frequently with hypopyon.*
- *Retinitis* (**Fig. 3.29**).

- *Occlusive periphlebitis and periarteritis* (**Fig. 3.30**).

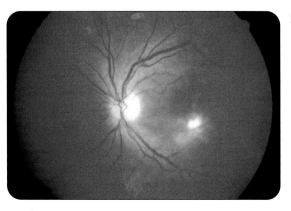

Fig. 3.29

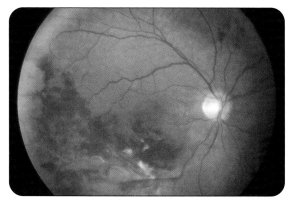

Fig. 3.30

CANDIDIASIS

- This may either be a localized mucocutaneous infection or a disseminated fungemia.
- Fungemia typically affects intravenous drug abusers, patients with long-term indwelling catheters and severely ill hospitalized patients who are also immunocompromised.
- Ocular involvement may occur with disseminated disease.

Systemic features

 Presentation

- Fever and other constitutional symptoms.

 Signs

- Multiple organ involvement, most commonly, renal, cerebral and cardiac.

Eye signs

- *Multifocal choroiditis.*
- *Vitreous 'cotton ball' colonies* (**Fig. 3.31**).
- Endophthalmitis and retinal necrosis in very severe cases.
- Roth spots and retinal hemorrhages.
- Anterior uveitis.

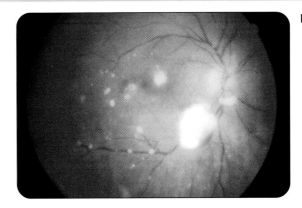

Fig. 3.31

CAROTID ARTERY STENOSIS

- This is a common atheromatous narrowing and ulceration involving the bifurcation of the common carotid artery in the neck into internal and external carotid arteries. **Fig. 3.32** shows minor right stenosis and complete left occlusion.
- The irregularity of the vessel wall may be the source of cerebral and retinal emboli composed of platelets and fibrin (white emboli) or tiny fragments of atheromatous material (Hollenhorst plaques).
- Ocular manifestations are frequent and may be the presenting feature.

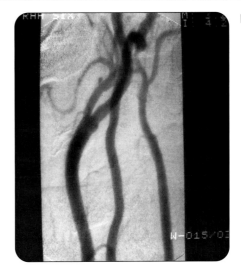

Fig. 3.32

Systemic features

 Presentation

- Transient retinal ischemic attacks (amaurosis fugax).
- Transient cerebral ischemic attacks.
- Stroke.

 Signs

- Diminished or absent pulsation of the involved cervical carotid arteries if the stenosis is severe.
- A bruit over the stenosis which is best heard with the bell of the stethoscope.

Eye signs

- *Asymptomatic Hollenhorst plaques.*
- Fibrinoplatelet emboli are seldom seen unless the patient is examined during an attack of amaurosis fugax.

- Retinal artery occlusion.
- Ocular ischemic syndrome.

CHANCROID

- This is a rare acute sexually transmitted disease that is endemic in areas of Africa and Asia caused by *Haemophilus ducreyi*.

- Ocular manifestations are infrequent.

Systemic features

- Painful genital ulceration.

- Inguinal lymphadenopathy which may become suppurated.

Eye signs

- Parinaud oculoglandular fever.

CHARCOT–MARIE–TOOTH DISEASE (PERONEAL MUSCULAR ATROPHY)

- This is a rare motor and sensory neuropathy initially involving the lower legs and later the small muscles of the hands.

- Inheritance is autosomal dominant or X-linked recessive.
- Ocular manifestations are infrequent.

Systemic features

 Presentation

- In childhood or adolescence with difficulties in walking or because of deformity of feet (pes cavus).

 Signs

- Progressive wasting of muscles below the knees giving rise to a 'stork leg' appearance (**Fig. 3.36**).
- Foot drop and a 'steppage' gait.
- Weakness and wasting of the small muscles of the hand.
- Sensory loss and diminished tendon reflexes.

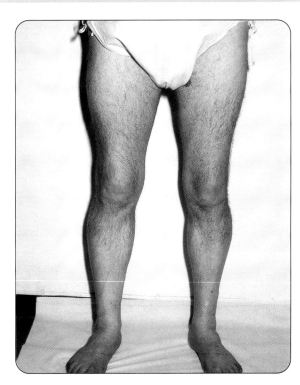

Fig. 3.36

Eye signs

- Optic atrophy.

CHÉDIAK–HIGASHI SYNDROME

- This is a very rare life-threatening condition which is associated with partial oculocutaneous albinism.

- Inheritance is autosomal recessive.

Systemic features

 Presentation

- In childhood with recurrent pyogenic infections due to a leukocyte killing defect.

 Signs

- Lymphadenopathy and hepatomegaly.

 Complications

- Early demise as a result of infection or lymphoma.

Eye signs

- *Ocular albinism.*

- Predisposition to retinal detachment.

CHLAMYDIAL GENITAL INFECTION

- This is a common sexually transmitted disease caused by D–K serotypes of *Chlamydia trachomatis*.

- Ocular manifestations are infrequent.

Systemic features

 Presentation

- In males with 'non-specific urethritis'.
- In females with abacterial pyuria and cervicitis.

 Complications

- In males epididymitis and it may trigger Reiter syndrome.
- In females it may result in infertility from chronic salpingitis.

Eye signs

- *Follicular conjunctivitis with mucopurulent discharge.*
- *Peripheral subepithelial corneal infiltrates* (**Fig. 3.37**).
- Superior corneal micropannus.

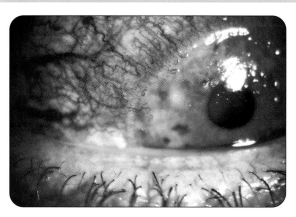

Fig. 3.37

CHURG–STRAUSS SYNDROME (ALLERGIC GRANULOMATOSIS)

- This is an uncommon multisystem disease characterized by the diagnostic triad of asthma, eosinophilia and systemic vasculitis.

- Ocular manifestations are infrequent.

Systemic features

 Presentation

- In the fourth decade.

 Signs

- Pulmonary hilar adenopathy and infiltrates (Löffler syndrome).

- Cutaneous vasculitis and subcutaneous nodules.
- Heart disease and hypertension.
- Arthralgia.
- Multifocal neuropathy.
- Glomerulonephritis.

Eye signs

- Scleritis.

- Retinal periarteritis.

CICATRICIAL PEMPHIGOID

- This is an uncommon, chronic autoimmune (type 2 hypersensitivity) disease characterized by recurrent sub-basal blisters of the mucous membranes and skin.

- It affects women more commonly than men.
- Ocular manifestations are very frequent and serious.

Systemic features

 Presentation

- In late middle age with ocular or mucocutaneous lesions or both.

 Signs

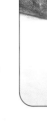
Fig. 3.38

- Mucosal blisters involving the mouth, nose, larynx, esophagus, anus, vagina and glans penis.
- Chronic skin blisters usually in the groins and extremities (**Fig. 3.38**) are usully sparse and heal by scarring.

Complications

- Scarring and stricture formation.

Eye signs

- *Severe cicatrizing conjunctivitis* (**Fig. 3.39**).

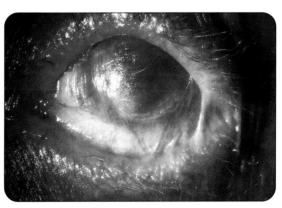
Fig. 3.39

CIRRHOSIS – PRIMARY BILIARY

- This is a rare, chronic, probably autoimmune, inflammatory, cholestatic liver disease which typically affects women.

- Ocular manifestations are infrequent.

147

Systemic features

 Presentation

- In the fifth decade with fatigue and hepatomegaly which may not be associated with signs of liver disease.

 Signs

- Jaundice, skin scratch marks, spider nevi and palmar erythema.

- White nails (leukonychia).
- Hepatosplenomegaly.

 Complications

- Secondary hypercholesterolemia with the formation of xanthelasma and tuberous lesions on extensor surfaces.
- Liver failure and gastrointestinal bleeding.

Eye signs

- Keratoconjunctivitis sicca.

COCCIDIOIDOMYCOSIS

- This is a rare infectious disease caused by the dimorphic fungus *Coccidioides immitis* which is found in north, central and south America.

- Ocular manifestations are infrequent.

Systemic features

 Presentation

- Acute self-limiting pulmonary 'flu-like' illness.
- Chronic but mild pulmonary infection.

 Signs

- Extrapulmonary lesions – erythema nodosum, arthropathy and meningitis.

Eye signs

- *Multifocal choroiditis* (**Fig. 3.40**).
- Anterior uveitis.

- Phlyctenular conjunctivitis (**Fig. 3.41**).

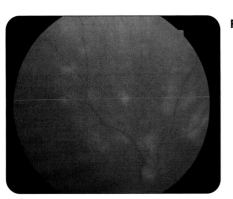

Fig. 3.40

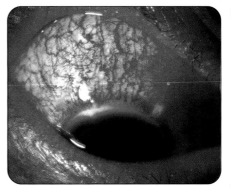

Fig. 3.41

COGAN SYNDROME

- This is a rare condition which is occasionally associated with polyarteritis nodosa.

- Ocular manifestations are frequent.

Systemic features

- Acute-onset of tinnitus, vertigo and deafness.

Eye signs

- Interstitial keratitis (**Fig. 3.42**).

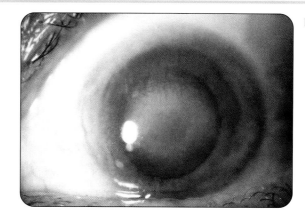

Fig. 3.42

CROHN DISEASE

- This is a common, idiopathic, chronic, relapsing, disease characterized by multifocal non-caseating granulomatous inflammation involving the full-thickness of the bowel (**Fig. 3.43**).
- It most frequently involves the ilcocecal region (**Fig. 3.44**), but any area of the bowel and even the mouth may be affected.
- Ocular manifestations are many but infrequent.

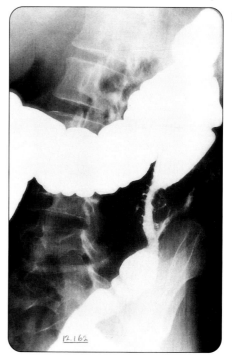

Fig. 3.44

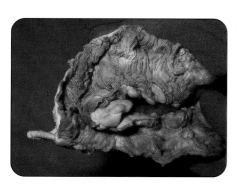

Fig. 3.43

Systemic features

 Presentation

- Usually in adult life but may be in childhood with fever, weight loss, diarrhea and abdominal pain.

 Signs

- Glossitis and aphthous mouth ulceration.
- Erythema nodosum.
- Pyoderma gangrenosum.
- Finger clubbing.

 Associations

- Acute peripheral arthritis, sacroiliitis and occasionally ankylosing spondylitis.

 Complications

- Obstruction due to stricture formation in the small or large intestine.
- Perirectal fistulae, abscesses and fissures.
- Occasionally sclerosing cholangitis.

Eye signs

- *Acute anterior uveitis.*
- *Conjunctivitis.*
- Peripheral corneal infiltrates.
- Retinal periphlebitis.

CRYPTOCOCCOSIS

- This is a rare systemic infection caused by a yeast *Cryptococcus neoformans*.
- The primary portal of entry is usually lung with subsequent spread to other sites.
- Patients with AIDS are particularly vulnerable.
- Ocular manifestations are infrequent.

Systemic features

 Presentation

- Usually with acute or subacute pulmonary symptoms.

 Signs

- Well-circumscribed areas of pulmonary infiltration.
- Disseminated disease is frequently the presenting feature in AIDS patients.

Eye signs

- *Multifocal choroiditis.*

CUSHING SYNDROME

- This rare condition is characterized by clinical features associated with prolonged elevation of free plasma glucocorticoid levels which may occur in the following three settings:

a. Systemic administration of corticosteroids.
b. Hypersecretion of glucocorticoids by the adrenal glands.
c. Hypersecretion of ACTH by a pituitary basophil adenoma (Cushing disease).
- Ocular manifestations are infrequent.

Systemic features

 Signs

- Obesity which may be trunkal or generalized.
- Plethora, moonface (**Fig. 3.45**), hirsutism (**Fig. 3.46**) and loss of scalp hair.
- Skin hyperpigmentation, striae (**Fig. 3.47**) and bruising.

- Muscle weakness, back pain and ankle edema.

 Complications

- Hypertension and diabetes.

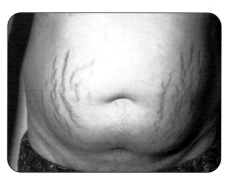

Fig. 3.47

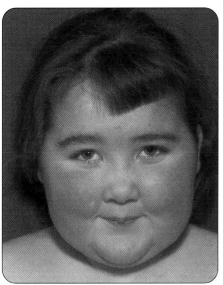

Fig. 3.45

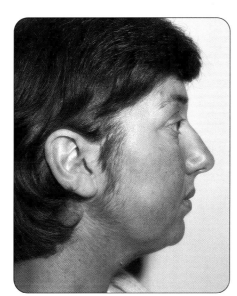

Fig. 3.46

Eye signs

- *Posterior subcapsular steroid-induced cataracts* (**Fig. 3.48**).
- Proptosis.
- Bitemporal hemianopia.

Fig. 3.48

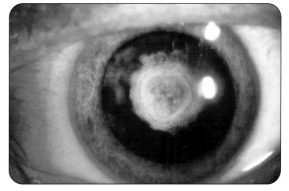

CYSTINOSIS

- This is a hereditary inborn error of amino acid metabolism which results from defective carrier-mediated transport of cystine through the lysosomal membrane and accumulation of cystine in the proximal renal tubules (Fanconi syndrome).
- Ocular manifestations are frequent and can be serious.
- The three types of cystinosis are as follows:

Infantile nephropathic cystinosis

Inheritance
- Autosomal recessive

 Presentation

- Poor feeding and failure to thrive associated with polyuria and thirst and other metabolic dysfunction due to proximal renal tubular acidosis.

 Systemic features

- Progressive renal dysfunction resulting in uremia by 10 years of age.
- Blond hair and fair complexion.
- Late sexual development but normal intellect.
- Hypothyroidism (**Fig. 3.49**).

 Eye signs

- Symptomatic corneal crystals in infancy (**Fig. 3.50**).
- Pigmentary retinopathy.

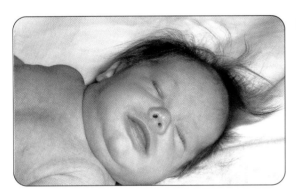
Fig. 3.49

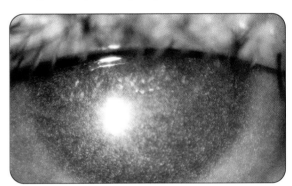
Fig. 3.50

Non-nephropathic cystinosis (formerly adult type)

Inheritance
- Autosomal dominant.

 Systemic features

- Normal renal function.

 Eye signs

- Asymptomatic corneal crystals.

Intermediate cystinosis (adolescent)

Inheritance
- Autosomal recessive.

 Systemic features

- Variable nephropathy.

 Eye signs

- Corneal crystals.

DERMATITIS HERPETIFORMIS

- This is an uncommon, chronic bullous dermatosis associated with gluten enteropathy.

- Ocular manifestations are infrequent.

Systemic features

 Presentation

- In the third or fourth decades.

 Signs

- Symmetrically distributed, small, itching skin blisters on an urticarial background.

Eye signs

- Cicatrizing conjunctivitis.

DERMATOMYOSITIS–POLYMYOSITIS

- This is an uncommon autoimmune disease characterized by combined degenerative and inflammatory changes in skeletal muscle.

- Mucocutaneous involvement occurs in dermatomyositis but not in polymyositis.
- Ocular manifestations are infrequent.

Systemic features

 Presentation

- At any time with a peak incidence in middle age in one of the following ways:
a. *Acute-onset disease* which is characterized by malaise, fever, widespread muscular pains and weakness which may involve the respiratory muscles and esophagus.
b. *Gradual-onset disease*, which is more common, is characterized by progressive muscular atrophy particularly of proximal limb muscles, without constitutional features.

 Signs

- Widespread erythematous skin rash on the face (**Fig. 3.51**), limbs and trunk (dermatomyositis).

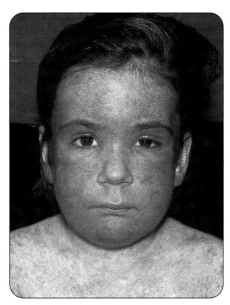

Fig. 3.51

- Subcutaneous calcification and ulceration over bony prominences may occur in children (**Fig. 3.52**).
- Acrosclerosis indistinguishable from scleroderma may involve the fingers (**Fig. 3.53**), face and chest wall.
- Raynaud phenomenon and nail fold thrombosis.

 Association

- High incidence of systemic malignancy, particularly bronchial carcinoma.

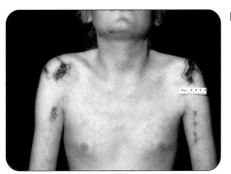

Fig. 3.52

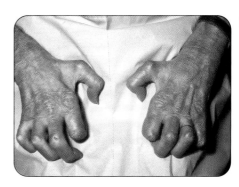

Fig. 3.53

Eye signs

- *Heliotrope periorbital erythema and edema* (**Fig. 3.54**).
- Retinal cotton-wool spots (**Fig. 3.55**).
- Keratoconjunctivitis sicca.

- Scleritis.
- Retinal periarteritis.

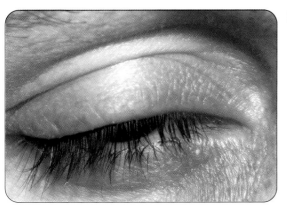

Fig. 3.54

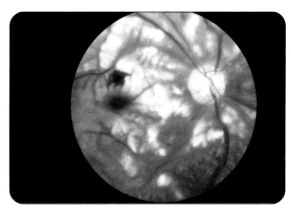

Fig. 3.55

DEVIC DISEASE (NEUROMYELITIS OPTICA)

- This is a rare disease characterized by simultaneous or sequential demyelination of the anterior visual pathways and spinal cord.

- Ocular manifestations are frequent and vision-threatening.

Systemic features

- Transverse myelitis and paraplegia.

Eye signs

- Bilateral retrobulbar neuritis with variable recovery.

DIABETES MELLITUS

- This is a common metabolic disease characterized by sustained hyperglycemia of varying severity secondary to lack of or diminished efficacy of endogenous insulin.

- The two main types are insulin dependent (type 1, juvenile-onset) and non-insulin dependent (type 2, maturity-onset).
- Ocular manifestations are frequent and serious.

Systemic features

 Presentation

- At any age in the following ways:
a. Acute-onset with weight loss polyuria, polydipsia and nocturia.
b. Gradual-onset with infections of the skin (**Fig. 3.56**), vulva (**Fig. 3.57**) or glans penis.

c. It may be asymptomatic and diagnosed by finding a fasting blood glucose concentration equal to or greater than 7.0 mmol/l or a random blood glucose concentration equal to or greater than 11.1 mmol/l.

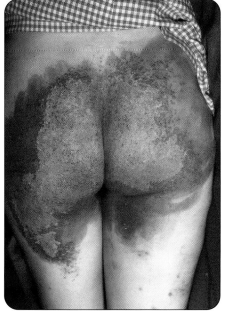

Fig. 3.56

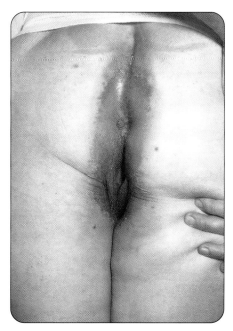

Fig. 3.57

Chronic complications

- Nephropathy.
- Accelerated atherosclerosis of the coronary and lower limb arteries.
- Polyneuropathy which is most frequently sensory and involves the feet.
- Blistering of the feet (**Fig. 3.58**).
- Painless, neuropathic perforating ulcers of the feet located at pressure points (**Fig. 3.59**).

- Painful, ischemic ulceration often located at the extremities.
- Gangrene of extremitis which may require amputation (**Fig. 3.60**).
- Neuropathic (Charcot) degenerative joint changes (**Fig. 3.61**).
- Necrobiosis lipoidica (**Fig. 3.62**).
- Lipodystrophy at sites of insulin injection (**Fig. 3.63**).
- Granuloma annulare.
- Diabetic mothers tend to produce large babies (**Fig. 3.64**).

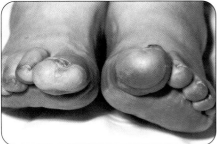

Fig. 3.58

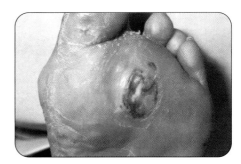

Fig. 3.59

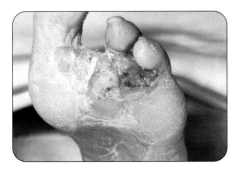

Fig. 3.60

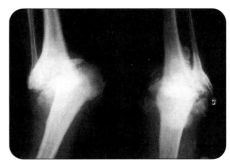

Fig. 3.61

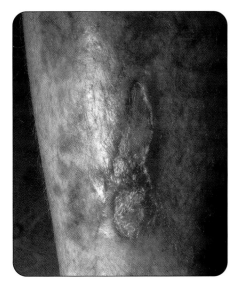

Fig. 3.62

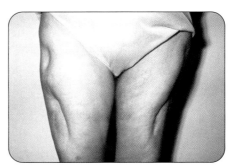

Fig. 3.63

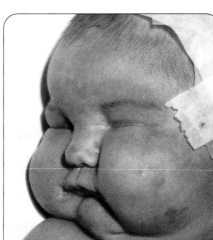

Fig. 3.64

Eye signs

- Retinopathy:
a. Background (**Fig. 3.65**).
b. Pre-proliferative (**Fig. 3.66**).
c. Proliferative (**Fig. 3.67**).
- Ocular motor nerve palsies (**Fig. 3.68**).
- Accelerated senile cataract.
- Acute early-onset cataract.

- Changes in refraction.
- Increased incidence of primary-open angle glaucoma.
- Papillopathy.
- Light–near dissociation of pupillary reactions.
- Iridopathy with increased iris transillumination.
- Asteroid hyalosis.
- Rhino-orbital mucormycosis.

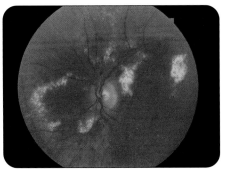

Fig. 3.65

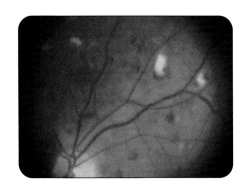

Fig. 3.66

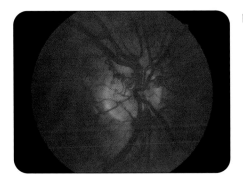

Fig. 3.67

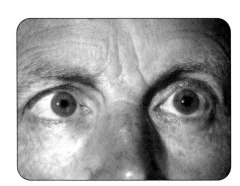

Fig. 3.68

DOWN SYNDROME

- This is a common, congenital chromosomal anomaly (trisomy for part or all of chromosome 21) the incidence of which is related to increased maternal age.

- Ocular manifestations are frequent but mainly innocuous.

Systemic features

 Signs

- Mental retardation and stunted growth.
- Round, flat face, small nose, small ears and protruding and fissured tongue (**Fig. 3.69**).
- Excess skin at the back of the neck.
- Hypotonia and protruberant abdomen.

- Short arms and legs.
- Small hands and fingers with a single transverse palmar (simian) crease.
- Congenital cardiac anomalies which may result in cyanosis and clubbing of the fingers (**Fig. 3.70**).
- Recurrent respiratory infections.

Eye signs

- *High myopia and retinal detachment* (**Fig. 3.75**).
- *Ocular fragility to trauma.*
- Lens subluxation.
- Keratoconus.
- Blue sclera.
- Angioid streaks.

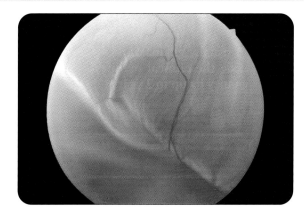

Fig. 3.75

EPIDERMOLYSIS BULLOSA

- This is a group of rare, inherited diseases characterized by the production of skin blisters following minor trauma.

- It is associated with a deficiency in collagen type 7 in the dermis.
- The incidence of ocular manifestations varies according the subgroup.

Subgroups and inheritance

a. Dominant simplex.
b. Recessive intermediate.

c. Dominant dystrophic.
d. Recessive dytrophic.

Systemic features

 Presentation

- During the neonatal period.

 Signs

- Chronic blistering and scarring of skin following minor skin trauma (**Fig. 3.76**).
- Mucosal involvement.
- Nail dystrophy.

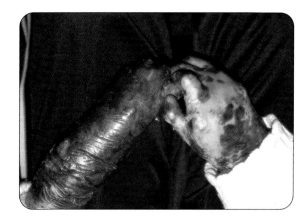

Fig. 3.76

Associations

- Increased risk of carcind
  less frequently of the du

- Multiple, frequently bi
  hypertrophy of the ret

- This is a common gra
  aorta and its major
  branches of the carot

Presentation

- In old age with a cc
  cation, anorexia, he
- Associated constit
  malaise, night swea
- Polymyalgia rheum
  follow the developn
- Unilateral or occasi
  presenting feature

Signs

- Tender thickened s
- Loss of arterial pul
- Ischemic necrosis

Complications

- Myocardial ischer
- Peripheral neurop
- Aortic aneurysm
- Brainsteam strok
  vertebral artery ir

! Complications

- Involvement of the esophagus which may lead to stenosis.
- Mitten-like scarring of hands and feet with partial syndactyly (Fig. 3.77).

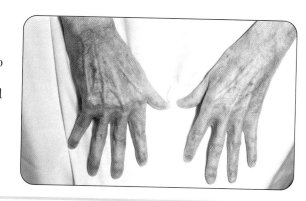

Fig. 3.77

Eye signs

These are most common in recessive dystrophic and least common in dominant simplex.
- *Corneal erosions.*
- *Scarring of eyelids.*
- Cicatrizing conjunctivitis.

FABRY DISEASE (ANGIOKERATOMA DIFFUSUM)

- This is a rare, lysosomal storage disease caused by deficiency of alpha-galactosidase with deposition of ceremide trihexoside in the kidneys, myocardium, cornea, peripheral and autonomic nerves.
- Inheritance is X-linked recessive.
- Ocular manifestations are many and frequent, some of which may be serious.

Systemic features

Presentation

- In childhood or adolescence with attacks of severe burning pain and paresthesiae involving the extremities which may be precipitated by heat, cold or physical exertion.

Signs

- Purple telangiectatic skin lesions (angiokeratomas) which are most numerous on the lower trunk and thighs.
- Cardiovascular, renal and pulmonary disease.
- Peripheral neuropathy.

Eye signs

- *Vortex keratopathy which is also present in female carriers* (Fig. 3.78).
- *Conjunctival telangiectasia.*
- *Congenital wedge-shaped cataracts* (Fig. 3.79).

- Retinal vascular tortosity, especially venous.
- Eyelid oedema.
- Third nerve palsy and nystagmus.

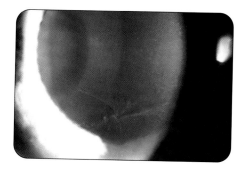

Fig. 3.78

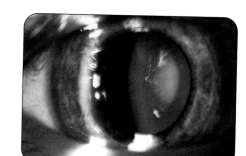

Fig. 3.79

Eye signs

- Anterior ischemic optic neuropathy which may be bilateral (**Fig. 3.83**).
- Cilioretinal artery occlusion.
- Cotton wool spots.
- Amaurosis fugax which often precedes visual loss.
- Third nerve palsy (sparing the pupil) and occasionally fourth or sixth nerve palsies.
- Ocular ischemic syndrome.

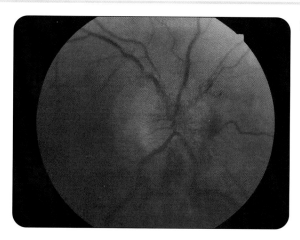

Fig. 3.83

- This is a rare here
- Inheritance is aut

Presentation

- During childhood

Signs

- Progressive ataxi
- Foot deformity (I
- Spinal deformity
- Dysarthria.
- Sensorineural de

Associations

- Cardiomyopathy
- Diabetes.

- *Pigmentary reti*
- *Nystagmus.*

- This is a rare intestinal poly
- Inheritance is

Signs

- Asymptomati colon, rectum and often tho

GONORRHEA

- This is an uncommon venereal genitourinary tract infection caused by a Gram-negative diplococcus *Neisseria gonorrhoeae*.

- Ocular manifestations are infrequent but serious.

Systemic features

In males
- Urethral discharge with dysuria of varying severity after about a 6-day incubation period.
- Urethral stricture formation is now an uncommon complication.

In females
- The infection is asymptomatic in 50% of cases.
- Symptomatic patients develop a vaginal discharge and less frequently dysuria.
- Untreated infection may ascend to the genital tract and cause chronic pelvic inflammatory disease.

Eye signs

- Hyperacute conjunctivitis with extremely profuse and thick creamy discharge (**Fig. 3.84**).

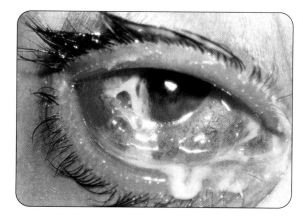

Fig. 3.84

GOODPASTURE SYNDROME

- This is a rare, rapidly progressive disease caused by linear deposition of anti-basement membrane antibodies along basement membranes of the kidneys and lungs.

- Ocular manifestations are infrequent and usually innocuous.

Systemic features

 Presentation

- Most frequently during the third decade and again in the sixth and seventh decades with malaise, hemoptysis, dyspnea, cough and renal manifestations.

 Signs

- Pulmonary inflammation.
- Glomerulonephritis and renal failure.

Eye signs

- Retinal hemorrhages and cotton-wool spots.
- Exudative retinal detachment.

GOUT

- This is a group of common metabolic disorders characterized by the deposition in tissues of monosodium urate monohydrate from hyperuricemic body fluids.

- Ocular manifestations are infrequent.

Systemic features

 Presentation

- Usually during the fourth or fifth decades with acute, usually monoarticular arthritis of a big toe, ankle, knee or finger.

 Complications

- Nephrolithiasis, urolithiasis and chronic renal disease.
- Hypertension.

 Signs

- Chronic, erosive, deforming arthritis associated with periarticular and subcutaneous urate deposits (tophi) is uncommon.

Eye signs

- Corneal crystals.

- Band keratopathy.

HEMOCHROMATOSIS – PRIMARY

- This is a rare multisystem disease in which iron in the body is increased and is deposited in various organs with damaging effects.

- Inheritance is autosomal recessive.
- Ocular manifestations are infrequent and innocuous.

Systemic features

 Presentation

- In adult life.

 Signs

- Heptomegaly.
- Skin hyperpigmentation.
- Cardiomyopathy.
- Arthropathy.
- Diabetes.

 Complications

- Cirrhosis, when present, is associated with an increased risk of hepatic carcinoma (**Fig. 3.85**).

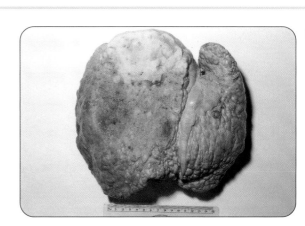

Fig. 3.85

Eye signs

- Keratoconjunctivitis sicca.

HERMANSKY–PUDLAK SYNDROME

- This is a very rare lysosomal storage disease of the reticuloendothelial system which is associated with platelet dysfunction.

- It is associated with tyrosinase-positive oculocutaneous albinism.
- Inheritance is autosomal recessive.

Systemic features

- Easy bruising, especially after aspirin ingestion.

- Pulmonary fibrosis.

Eye signs

- *Ocular albinism.*

HISTIOCYTOSIS X (LANGERHANS CELL HISTIOCYTOSIS)

- This is group of three clinically different conditions in which multiple infiltrative foci of histiocytes occur that bear features of Langerhans cells.

- The incidence of ocular manifestations varies according to the subgroup.

Eosinophilic granuloma

 Systemic features

- Mainly pulmonary and bone involvement.

 Eye signs

- Occasional proptosis.

Letterer–Siwe disease

 Systemic features

- Usually fatal in infancy with involvement of skin, lymph nodes, liver, spleen and bones.

 Eye signs

- Rarely proptosis.

Hand–Schüller–Christian disease

 Systemic features

- Bone lesions and diabetes insipidus.
- Pulmonary involvement with hilar lymphadenopathy.

 Eye signs

- Frequently proptosis (**Fig. 3.86**).

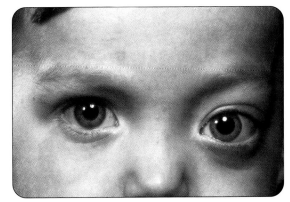

Fig. 3.86

HISTOPLASMOSIS

- This is a systemic fungal infection caused by *Histoplasma capsulatum*.

- Ocular manifestations are infrequent but serious.

Systemic features

 Presentation

- Asymptomatic infection is by far the most common and the only evidence is a positive skin test. The vast majority of patients with eye involvement fall into this group.

- Acute pulmonary involvement characterized by pyrexia, malaise, cough and hilar lymphadenopathy is much less common.
- Other types are chronic pulmonary and disseminated, the latter may be seen in patients with AIDS.

Eye signs

- Multifocal choroiditis associated with peripapillary atrophy.
- Secondary choroidal neovascularization and hemorrhage at the macula (**Fig. 3.87**).

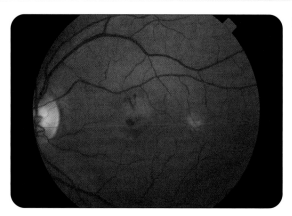

Fig. 3.87

HOMOCYSTINURIA

- This is a rare, disorder of amino acid metabolism in which deficiency of cystathione beta-synthase leading to accumulation of homocystine and methionine.

- The condition is phenotypically similar to Marfan syndrome but with a thrombotic tendency.
- Inheritance is autosomal recessive.
- Ocular manifestations are frequent and serious.

Systemic features

 Signs

- Blond hair and a malar flush.
- Marfanoid habitus.
- Arachnodactyly is infrequent.
- Mental retardation and psychiatric disturbance.

 Complications

- Osteoporosis and spontaneous crush fractures.
- Seizures and small brain infarcts.
- Thromboses which may occur in any vessel and at any age.
- Postoperative and postpartum risk of thrombosis is high.

Eye signs

- *Downward lens subluxation.*

- *Myopia and retinal detachment.*

HYPERLIPOPROTEINEMIAS

- This is a group of disorders in which there is increased in levels of circulating lipoprotein.

- Hyperlipoproteinemia may be either primary or secondary to some other disease such as diabetes, thyroid disease or hepatic dysfunction.
- Ocular manifestations are frequent.

Classification of primary hyperlipoproteinemia

- Type II a in which only cholesterol is elevated to exceed 6.5 mmol/l.

- Type II b in which both cholesterol and triglycerides are elevated.

Systemic features

 Signs

- Tendon xanthomata.

 Complications

- Atherosclerosis and coronary artery disease.

Eye signs

- *Xanthelasma of the eyelids.*
- *Corneal arcus.*
- Retinal vein occlusion.
- Lipemia retinalis (**Fig. 3.88**).

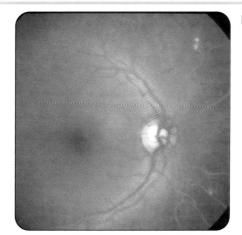

Fig. 3.88

HYPERLYSINEMIA

- This is a rare, inborn error of amino acid metabolism associated with deficiency of lysine alpha-ketoglutarate reductase.

- Inheritance is autosomal recessive.
- Ocular manifestations are infrequent.

Systemic features

 Signs

- Mental retardation.

- Lax ligaments and hypotonic muscles.
- Seizures.

Eye signs

- Microspherophakia (**Fig. 3.89**).
- Ectopia lentis.

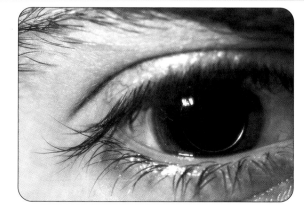
Fig. 3.89

HYPERORNITHINEMIA

- This is a rare, inborn error of ornithine metabolism associated with deficiency of ornithine aminotransferase.

- Inheritance is autosomal recessive.
- Ocular manifestations are universal and serious.

Systemic features

 Presentation

- In childhood or early teens with the onset of myopia.

 Signs

- Hyperornithinemia.
- Ornithinuria.

Eye signs

- *Gyrate atrophy of the retina and choroid* (**Fig. 3.90**).
- Early-onset cataracts.

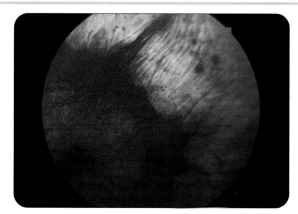
Fig. 3.90

HYPERPARTHYROIDISM – PRIMARY

- This is caused by oversecretion of parathyroid hormone which results in hypercalcemia.

- The most common cause is a single parathyroid adenoma and a minority of cases are caused by diffuse hyperplasia.

Systemic features

 Presentation

- Usually in middle age with renal calculi.

 Signs

- Bone disease (osteitis fibrosa cystica).
- Hypotonicity of muscles and ligaments.
- Gastrointestinal disease.
- Neurological problems.

Eye signs

- Band keratopathy.

HYPERTENSION

- This is most commonly idiopathic (essential) and occasionally secondary to a renal or metabolic disorder.

- Ocular manifestations are frequent but usually non-sight-threatening.

Systemic features

 Presentation

- Usually in adult life.
- In the absence of complications there are no symptoms.

 Signs

- Blood pressure in excess of 140/90.

Complications

- Left ventricular hypertrophy and left ventricular failure.
- Increased risk of atherosclerosis resulting in coronary heart disease and stroke.
- Renal disease.

Eye signs

- *Retinopathy:*
a. Arteriolar attenuation and constriction (**Fig. 3.91**).
b. Arteriolosclerosis (**Fig. 3.92**).
c. Hemorrhages, cotton-wool spots and a macular star (**Fig. 3.93**).
d. Disc edema (malignant phase) (**Fig. 3.94**).

- *Retinal vein occlusion.*
- *Non-arteritic anterior ischemic optic neuropathy.*
- Ocular motor nerve palsies.
- Retinal artery macroaneurysm (**Fig. 3.95**).
- Retinal artery occlusion.
- Exudative retinal detachment in eclampsia.

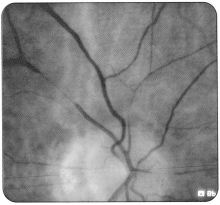

Fig. 3.91

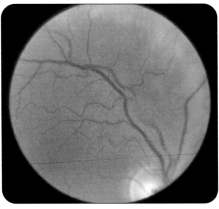

Fig. 3.92

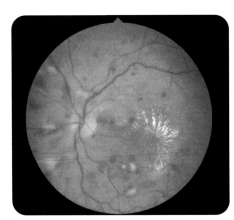

Fig. 3.93

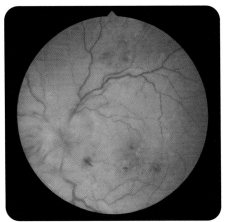

Fig. 3.94

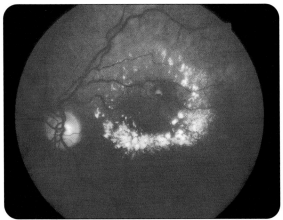

Fig. 3.95

ICHTHYOSIS – ACQUIRED

- This is an uncommon skin disease which is occasionally associated with an underlying systemic disease.

Systemic features

 Signs

- Itchy, dry and scaly skin which may be associated with hyperkeratosis.

 Associations

- Lymphoma.
- Refsum disease.

Eye signs

(*see* Lymphomas, p. 182 and Refsum disease, p. 207)

IgA NEPHROPATHY

- This is a common glomerulonephritis which affects males more commonly than females.

- Ocular manifestations are infrequent.

Systemic features

 Presentation

- Usually in the second or third decades with hematuria, pharyngitis, fever, lethargy and diffuse muscle pains.

 Complications

- The disease may be self-limiting or it may result in renal failure.

Eye signs

- Anterior uveitis.

JUVENILE IDIOPATHIC ARTHRITIS

- This is an uncommon sero-negative arthritis with an onset prior to the age of 16 years.
- Ocular manifestations are frequent and serious.

- Based on the onset and extent of joint involvement during the first 6 months, the three types of presentation are as follows:

173

Eye signs

- *Acute bilateral conjunctivitis* (**Fig. 3.101**).
- *Superficial punctate keratitis.*
- *Anterior uveitis.*
- Retinal periarteritis.

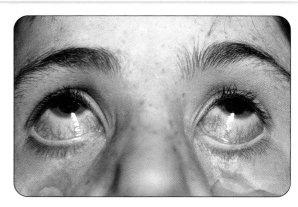

Fig. 3.101

KEARNS–SAYRE SYNDROME

- This is a rare mitochondrial cytopathy associated with mitochondrial DNA deletions.
- Ocular manifestations are universal.

Systemic features

 Presentation

- In childhood or adolescence with an insidious onset of bilateral ptosis and ophthalmoplegia.

 Signs

- Heart block.

- Ataxia.
- Proximal muscle weakness.
- Short stature.

 Associations

- Deafness, diabetes and hypoparathyroidism.

Eye signs

- *Ptosis* (**Fig. 3.102**).
- *Progressive, symmetrical external ophthalmoplegia.*
- *Pigmentary retinopathy.*

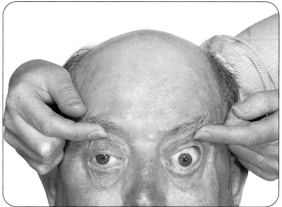

Fig. 3.102

KLIPPEL–TRENAUNAY–WEBER SYNDROME

- This is a rare congenital disorder characterized by cutaneous hemangiomas.

- Ocular manifestations are frequent.

Systemic features

 Signs

- Facial nevus flammeus (**Fig. 3.103**).
- Hemangiomas on legs, buttocks (**Fig. 3.104**), abdomen and lower trunk.

- Hypertrophy of usually one limb (**Fig. 3.105**).

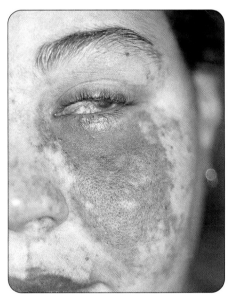

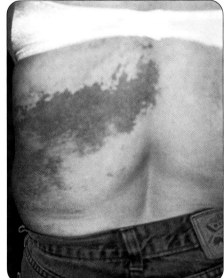

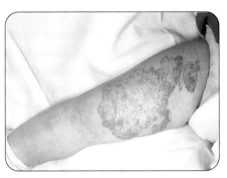

Fig. 3.105

Fig. 3.103

Fig. 3.104

Eye signs

- Glaucoma.
- Ocular hemangiomas.

- Orbital varices.

LECITHIN–CHOLESTEROL–ACETYLTRANSFERASE DEFICIENCY (NORUM DISEASE)

- This is a rare disorder of lipid metabolism in which there is accumulation of unesterified cholesterol.

- Inheritance is autosomal recessive.
- Ocular manifestations are frequent but innocuous.

Systemic features

 Presentation

- Early-onset atherosclerosis.

 Signs

- Renal disease.
- Anemia.

Eye signs

- Corneal arcus-like clouding.

LEPROSY (HANSEN DISEASE)

- This is a chronic granulomatous disease caused by the intracellular acid-fast bacillus *Mycobacterium leprae*.

- Ocular manifestations are frequent and serious.

Systemic signs

1. Lepromatous leprosy

 Signs

- Erythema nodosum.
- Thickening of nasal mucosa.
- Saddle-shaped nose.
- Cutaneous plaques and nodules (**Fig. 3.106**).
- Sensory neuropathy which may eventually result in trauma and shortening of digits.

2. Tuberculoid leprosy

 Signs

- Annular skin lesions with raised edges and hypopigmented centres.
- Thickening of cutaneous sensory nerves.
- Muscular wasting and contracture resulting in claw hand and claw toes.

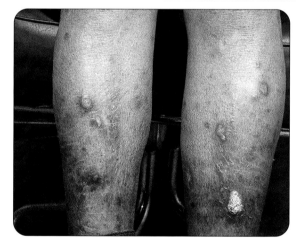

Fig. 3.106

Eye signs

- *Madarosis.*
- *Lagophthalmos secondary to seventh nerve palsy.*
- *Keratitis.*
- *Anterior uveitis.*
- Miosis (**Fig. 3.107**).

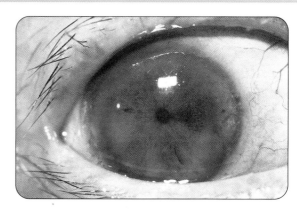

Fig. 3.107

LEUKEMIAS

- The leukemias are a group of uncommon malignancies of leukocytes.

- Ocular manifestations are frequent.

Classification

a. *Acute lymphoblastic* which typically affects children.
b. *Acute myeloid* which occurs more frequently in adults.

c. *Chronic leukemias* (myeloid and lymphatic), which typically affect the elderly.

Systemic features of acute leukemias

 Presentation

- A subacute onset of fatigue due to anemia and an increased tendency to bleed.

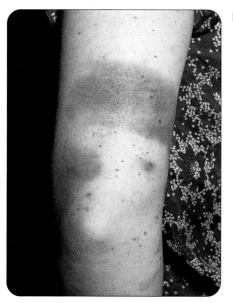

Fig. 3.108

 Signs

- Pallor of mucous membranes due to anemia.
- Purpura, easy bruising (**Fig. 3.108**) and bleeding (**Fig. 3.109**) due to thrombocytopenia.
- Infiltrative features include lymphadenopathy and splenomegaly.

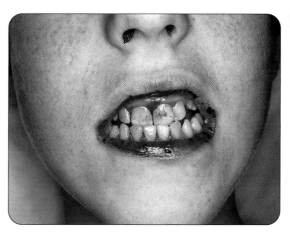

Fig. 3.109

Systemic features of chronic leukemias

 Presentation

- Insiduous onset of fatigue, weight loss and infection.
- In some cases the diagnosis may be made by chance.

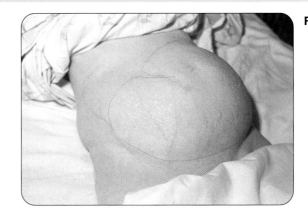
Fig. 3.110

▲ **Signs**

- Lymphadenopathy and splenomegaly (**Fig. 3.110**).

Eye signs

- The leukemias may involve almost any ocular tissue either by direct infiltration, or secondary manifestations such as anemia, thrombocytopenia, hyperviscosity and opportunistic infection.

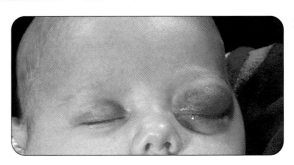
Fig. 3.111

Orbit
- This is occasionally involved, particularly in children with an extramedullary type of acute myeloid leukemia (**Fig. 3.111**).

Anterior segment
This most frequently occurs in patients with acute lymphoblastic leukemia.
- Spontaneous subconjunctival hemorrhage.
- Spontaneous hyphema (**Fig. 3.112**).
- Pseudo-hypopyon (**Fig. 3.113**).
- Iris infiltration and thickening.

Fundus
- Hemorrhages and Roth spots (**Fig. 3.114**).
- Peripheral retinal neovascularization in chronic myeloid leukemia.
- Choroidal infiltration may occur in all leukemias (**Fig. 3.115**).
- Optic neuropathy due to infiltration of the optic nerve head may occur in acute myeloid leukemia.

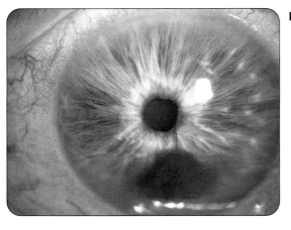
Fig. 3.112

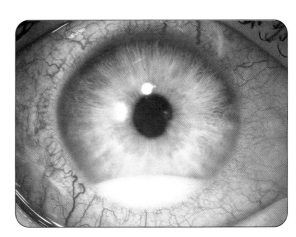
Fig. 3.113

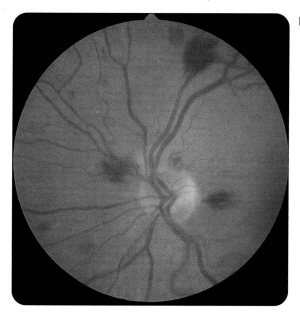

Fig. 3.114

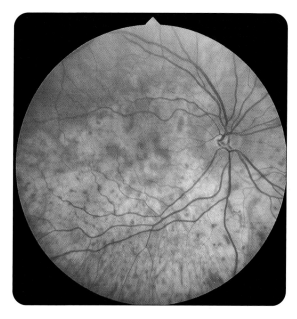

Fig. 3.115

LINEAR IgA DISEASE (BULLOUS DERMATOSIS)

- This is a rare blistering mucocutaneous disease.

- Ocular manifestations are frequent.

Systemic features

 Presentation

- In the fourth and fifth decades.

 Signs

- Frequent mucosal involvement.
- Tense skin blisters of varying size which are usually self-limiting.

Eye signs

- *Cicatrizing conjunctivitis.*

LYME DISEASE

- This uncommon condition is caused by *Borrelia burgdorferi* infection which is transmitted by the deer tick *Ixodes*.

- Ocular manifestations are frequent and may be serious.

Systemic features

 Signs

Stage 1
- Skin lesion (erythema chronica migrans).
- Flu-like symptoms and lymphadenopathy.

Stage 2
- Initially cranial nerve palsies and later predominantly peripheral neuropathy.

- Arthralgia.
- Myocarditis and dysrhythmia.

Stage 3
- Arthritis.
- Demyelinating encephalopathy.

Eye signs

Stage 1
- Conjunctivitis.

Stage 2
- Intermediate uveitis.
- Neuroretinitis.

Stage 3
- Interstitial keratitis.

LYMPHOGRANULOMA VENEREUM

- This is a rare sexually transmitted disease caused by infection with a strain of *Chlamydia trachomatis*.

- Ocular manifestations are infrequent.

Systemic features

 Presentation

- Painless genital ulceration.
- Painful regional lymphadenopathy.

- An acute form may present with proctitis which may be associated with perirectal abscess.

Eye signs

- Parinaud oculoglandular fever.

- Interstitial keratitis.

LYMPHOMAS

- This is group of uncommon diseases characterized by neoplastic proliferation of cells of the immune system.

- The incidence of ocular manifestations is related to the type of lymphoma.

Hodgkin disease

 Systemic features

- Asymptomatic lymphadenopathy.
- Fever, night sweats and weight loss.

 Eye signs

These are uncommon and are usually associated with advanced disease.
- Anterior uveitis.
- Vitritis.
- Multifocal fundus lesions resembling chorioretinitis.

Non-Hodgkin lymphoma

 Systemic features

- Asymptomatic lymphadenopathy.
- Weight loss and fever are less common than in Hodgkin disease.

 Eye signs

These are frequent.
- Proptosis which may be bilateral.
- Conjunctival lymphoma (**Fig. 3.116**).
- Mikulicz syndrome.
- Rarely uveal infiltration.

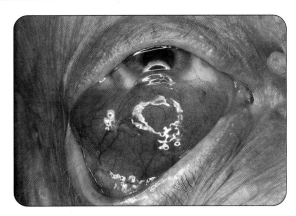

Fig. 3.116

Central nervous system B-cell lymphoma

 Systemic features

These usually develop after the onset of ocular involvement.
- Headache and focal signs caused by intracranial masses.
- Neuropathies caused by leptomeningeal infiltration.
- Bilateral motor and sensory signs affecting the limbs due to spinal cord disease.
- Systemic nodal or visceral lesions are uncommon.

 Eye signs

- *Granulomatous anterior uveitis.*
- *Intermediate uveitis.*
- *Multifocal, yellow, subpigment epithelial infiltrates.*
- Geographic encircling choroidal infiltration (**Fig. 3.117**).

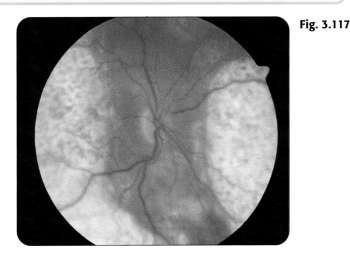

Fig. 3.117

MARFAN SYNDROME

- This is an uncommon disorder of connective tissue.
- Inheritance is autosomal dominant with variable expressivity.
- Ocular manifestations are frequent and serious.

Systemic features

 Signs

Skeletal
- Tall and thin stature.
- The limbs are disproportionately long as compared with the trunk (**Fig. 3.118**).
- Long and spider-like fingers (arachnodactyly) (**Fig. 3.119**).
- Mild joint hypermobility.
- Asymmetric anterior chest deformity with either depression (**Fig. 3.120**) or prominence of the sternum.
- A narrow and high-arched (gothic) palate.
- Scoliosis.

Cardiovascular
- Dilatation of the ascending aorta leading to aortic incompetence and dissection.
- Mitral valve disease.

Miscellaneous
- Muscular underdevelopment with a predisposition to hernias.
- Cutaneous striae, fragility and easy bruising.

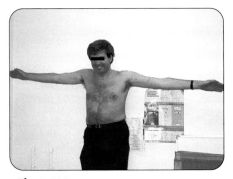

Fig. 3.118

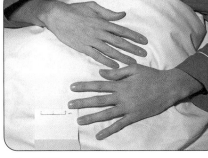

Fig. 3.119

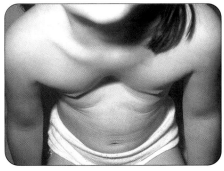

Fig. 3.120

Eye signs

Lens
- Ectopia lentis, which is bilateral, symmetrical, non-progressive and usually upwards (**Fig. 3.121**).
- Microspherophakia.

Cornea
- Megalocornea.
- Keratoconus.

Iris
- Hypoplasia of the dilator pupillae.
- Transillumination defects.

Glaucoma
- Associated with congenital angle anomaly.
- Secondary to lens subluxation.

Posterior segment
- High myopia.
- Lattice degeneration (**Fig. 3.122**).
- Retinal detachment.

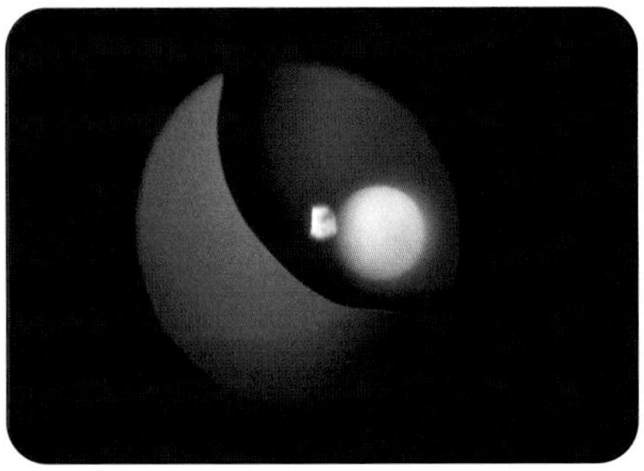

Fig. 3.121

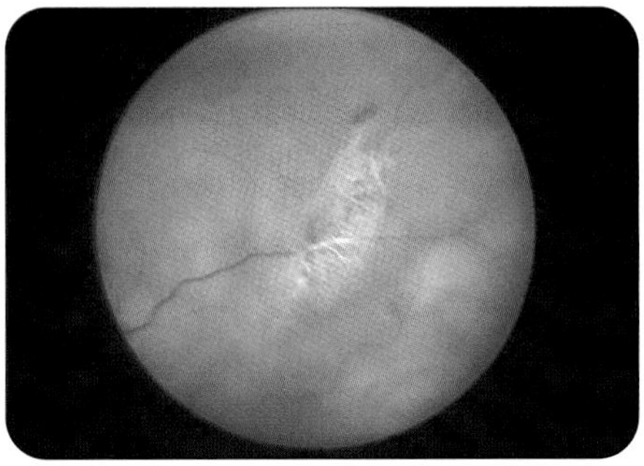

Fig. 3.122

MEMBRANOPROLIFERATIVE GLOMERULONEPHRITIS TYPE II

- This is an uncommon, idiopathic renal disorder with characteristic histologic features.

- Ocular manifestations are frequent but innocuous.

Systemic features

 Presentation

- In childhood with nephrotic syndrome or acute nephritis.

 Signs

- Renal impairment.
- Hypertension.

Eye signs

- Bilateral, diffuse, yellow drusen-like deposits at the posterior pole (**Fig. 3.123**).

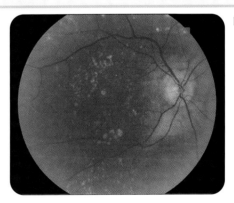

Fig. 3.123

MERETOJA SYNDROME

- This is a rare condition which is characterized by familial amyloidosis and corneal lattice dystrophy type 2.

- Inheritance is autosomal dominant.

Systemic features

 Signs

- Cranial nerve palsies with a predilection for the facial.
- Polyneuropathy.
- The facial expression is characteristic with a protruding lip and mask-like facies.
- Skin laxity.

Associations

- Renal and cardiac disease.

Eye signs

- *Corneal lattice distrophy type 2* (**Fig. 3.124**).
- Blepharochalasis.

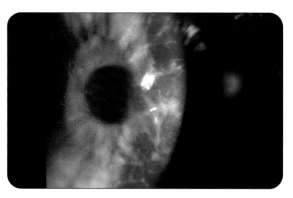

Fig. 3.124

MIXED CONNECTIVE TISSUE DISEASE

- This uncommon condition is characterized by clinical features of systemic lupus erythematosus, systemic sclerosis and polymyositis.

- Ocular manifestations are frequent.

Systemic features

 Signs

- Raynaud phenomenon.
- Arthritis.

- Esophageal hypomotility.
- Diminished pulmonary diffusion capacity.
- Inflammatory myopathy.

Eye signs

- *Keratoconjunctivitis sicca.*

MULTIPLE ENDOCRINE NEOPLASIA TYPE IIB (SIPPLE SYNDROME)

- This is a rare disease characterized by potentially lethal endocrine tumors.

- Inheritance is autosomal dominant with a high degree of penetrance.
- Ocular manifestations are frequent.

Systemic features

 Signs

- Thickened lips and tongue due to mucosal neuromas.
- Marfanoid habitus.

 Associations

- Medullary cell thyroid carcinoma (**Fig. 3.125**).
- Pheochromocytoma.
- Hyperparathyroidism.
- Intestinal ganglioneuromatosis.

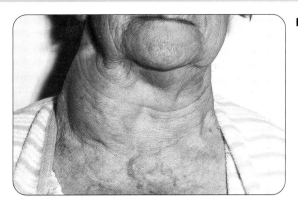

Fig. 3.125

Eye signs

- *Prominent corneal nerves.*
- *Neurofibromas of the eyelids.*

- Conjunctival neuromas.
- Impaired pupillary dilatation.

MULTIPLE MYELOMA (MYELOMATOSIS)

- This is an uncommon progressive disease caused by malignant plasma cell proliferation in bone marrow.

- Ocular manifestations are infrequent.

Systemic features

 Presentation

- In middle or old age with weakness and fatigue due to marrow failure.
- Backache due to osteoporosis or tumor invasion.

 Signs

- Osteolytic lesions and osteoporosis involving long bones (**Fig. 3.126**), the axial skeleton and the skull.
- Pathologic fractures of long bones and ribs may occur with advanced disease.

 Complications

- Hypercalcemia.
- Renal disease.
- Recurrent infections secondary to hypogammaglobulinemia.

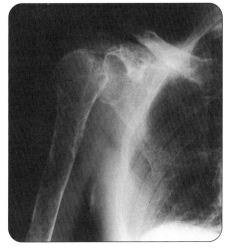

Fig. 3.126

Eye signs

- *Corneal crystals.*
- *Slow-flow retinopathy.*
- Retinal vein occlusion (**Fig. 3.127**).
- Proptosis.
- Pars plana cysts.

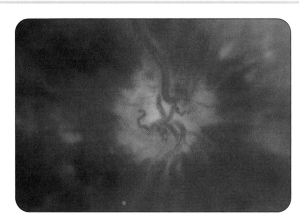

Fig. 3.127

MULTIPLE SCLEROSIS

- This is a common idiopathic, remitting disease involving white matter within the central nervous system.
- **Fig. 3.128** is an axial MRI scan (*left* T1-weighted, *right* T2-weighted) showing the characteristic periventicular location of plaques of demyelination.
- Ocular manifestations are frequent.

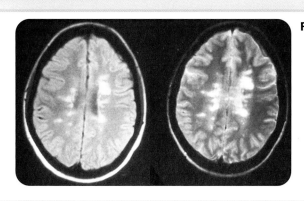

Fig. 3.128

Systemic features

Presentation

- Usually in early adult life with remitting/relapsing involvement occurring at random frequency and of unpredictable duration.

Signs

a. *Spinal cord lesions* resulting in weakness, stiffness and sphincter disturbance.
b. *Brainstem lesions* resulting in diplopia, nystagmus, dysarthria and dysphagia.
c. *Hemisphere lesions* resulting in hemiparesis, hemianopia and dysphasia.
d. *Other lesions* – tonic spasms and dysarthria–dysequilibrium–diplopia syndrome.

Eye signs

- *Retrobulbar neuritis.*
- *Internuclear ophthalmoplegia.*
- *Nystagmus.*
- Skew deviation.

- Ocular motor nerve palsies.
- Hemianopias.
- Intermediate uveitis.
- Retinal periphlebitis.

MYASTHENIA GRAVIS

- This is an uncommon autoimmune disease characterized by weakness of skeletal musculature due to impaired transmission at the neuromuscular junction.

- Ocular manifestations are very frequent.

Systemic features

 Presentation

- Most frequent in the third and fourth decades with diplopia, ptosis and excessive fatiguability of other muscles.

 Signs

- Weakness, particularly of the arms and proximal muscles of the legs, which increases with exercise.

- Lack of facial expression.
- Nasal speech, as well as difficulties in chewing and swallowing.
- Respiratory muscle involvement is rare but potentially serious.
- Exaggerated tendon reflexes with absence of sensory changes.
- Permanent myopathic wasting may occur in long-standing cases.

Eye signs

- *Ptosis which is bilateral but frequently asymmetrical* (**Fig. 3.129**).
- *Weakness of eyelid closure* (**Fig. 3.130**).

- *Cogan 'twitch' sign which is a brief upshoot of the eyelid on saccade from depression to the primary position.*
- *Diplopia which is frequently vertical.*
- Pseudo-internuclear ophthalmoplegia.

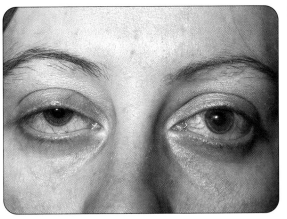

Fig. 3.129

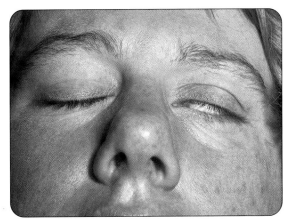

Fig. 3.130

MYOTONIC DYSTROPHY

- This is a rare disease characterized by myotonia which is the continued contraction of a muscle after cessation of voluntary effort.

- Inheritance is autosomal dominant with variable penetrance.
- Ocular manifestations are frequent.

Systemic features

Presentation

- Between the third and sixth decades with weakness of the hands and difficulty in walking.

Signs

- Myotonic peripheral muscle involvement which makes release of grip difficult.
- Mournful facial expression caused by bilateral facial wasting with hollow cheeks.
- Slurred speech from involvement of the tongue and pharyngeal muscles.
- Muscle wasting (**Fig. 3.131**).

Associations

- Frontal baldness in males.
- Hypogonadism.
- Hyperhidrosis.
- Intellectual deterioration.
- Pulmonary and cardiac disease.

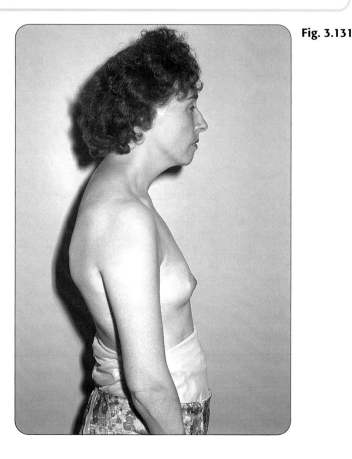

Fig. 3.131

Eye signs

- *Early-onset cataract.*
- *Ptosis.*
- *Light–near dissociation of pupillary reactions.*

- Symmetrical external ophthalmoplegia.
- Pigmentary retinopathy without visual impairment.
- Low intraocular pressure.

MYXEDEMA (HYPOTHYROIDISM)

- This is a common disease caused by thyroid hormone deficiency which may caused by primary thyroid dysfunction or from disorders affecting the hypo-thalamic–pituitary axis (secondary).

- Ocular manifestations are common but innocuous.

Systemic features

 Presentation

- At any age with an insidious onset of lethargy, weight gain, constipation, cold intolerance and a husky voice.

 Signs

General
- Goitre may be present in some patients.
- Puffy face (**Fig. 3.132**) and hands.
- Slow return of deep tendon reflexes.
- Deafness.
- Carpal tunnel syndrome.

Skin
- Alopecia (**Fig. 3.133**) and vitiligo.
- Dryness (**Fig. 3.134**).
- Pallor or a yellow color.
- Hirsutism in females.

Cardiovascular
- Bradycardia.
- Coronary artery disease.

Mental state
- Slowing, depression, poor memory, hypersomnescence and psychosis.

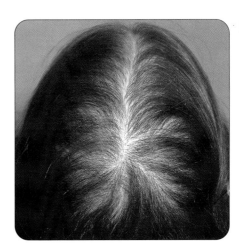
Fig. 3.133

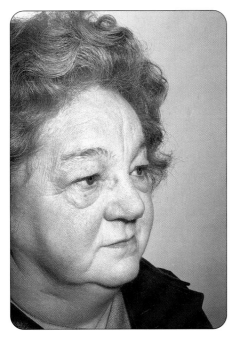
Fig. 3.132

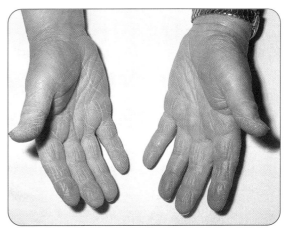
Fig. 3.134

Eye signs

- Madarosis.
- Puffiness of eyelids and periorbital skin (**Fig. 3.135**).
- Corneal arcus if plasma cholesterol is raised.

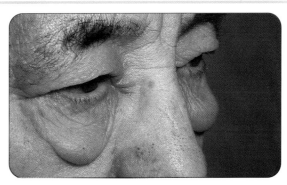
Fig. 3.135

NEUROFIBROMATOSIS–1 (VON RECKLINGHAUSEN DISEASE)

- This is a rare condition characterized by multiple neuronal tumors.
- Inheritance is autosomal dominant.
- Ocular manifestations are frequent.

Systemic features

 Signs

Neural
- Neural tumors which may involve the brain, peripheral nerves and autonomic nerves.
- Neurofibromas involving the mediastinum, pelvis or retro-abdomen.
- Epilepsy.

Skeletal
- Scoliosis.
- Congenital absence of greater wing of the sphenoid bone.
- Dysplasia or thinning of long bone cortex.
- Facial hemiatrophy and deformity (**Fig. 3.136**).
- Short stature.

Skin
- Café-au-lait spots (**Fig. 3.137**).
- Axillary and inguinal freckling.
- Nodular and pedunculated neurofibromas (**Fig. 3.138**).
- Plexiform neurofibromas (**Fig. 3.139**).

 Associations

- Malignant transformation of peripheral neurofibroma.
- Embryonal tumors of childhood.
- Hypertension which may be secondary to pheochromocytoma.
- Mental deterioration.

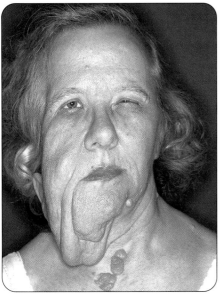

Fig. 3.136

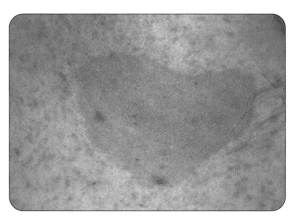

Fig. 3.137

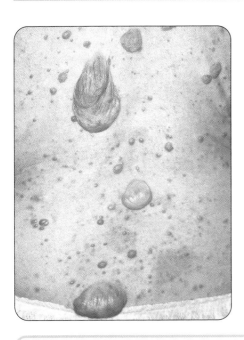

Fig. 3.138

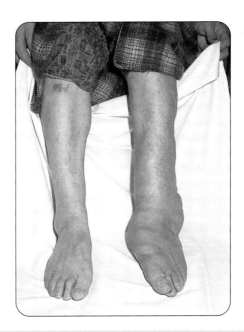

Fig. 3.139

Eye signs

- *Optic nerve glioma.*
- *Neural tumors of the orbit.*
- *Spheno-orbital encephalocele.*
- *Nodular eyelid neurofibromas.*
- *Plexiforn eyelid neurofibromas* (**Fig. 3.140**).
- *Lisch nodules* (**Fig. 3.141**).

- Congenital ectropion uveae (**Fig. 3.142**).
- Prominent corneal nerves.
- Glaucoma.
- Choroidal nevi which are multifocal and bilateral.
- Retinal astrocytomas.
- Choroidal neurofibromas.

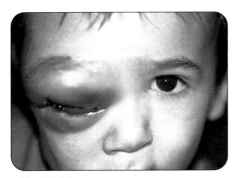

Fig. 3.140

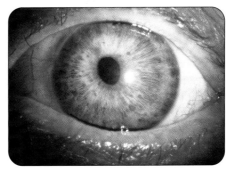

Fig. 3.141

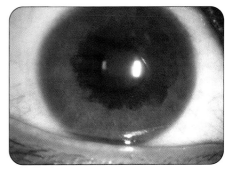

Fig. 3.142

NEUROFIBROMATOSIS-2

- This is less common than NF-1.
- Inheritance is autosomal dominant.

- Ocular manifestations are infrequent.

Systemic features

 Signs

- Bilateral vestibular schwannomas which develop during the second and third decades of life.

- Occasionally other CNS tumors such as neurofibromas, meningiomas, gliomas and schwannomas.

Eye signs

- *Early-onset cataracts.*
- Combined hamartomas of the retinal pigment epithelium and retina (**Fig. 3.143**).
- Extraocular motility defects.

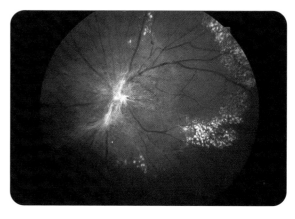

Fig. 3.143

NEVUS OF OTA

- This is a rare, congenital condition characterized by skin hyperpigmentation which typically affects Oriental females.

- Ocular manifestations are universal.

Systemic features

 Signs

- Unilateral hyperpigmentation of deep facial skin, most frequently in the distribution of the first and second divisions of the trigeminal nerve.
- Occasional involvement of the third division and of the nasal and buccal mucosa.

 Associations

- Rarely melanoma of the CNS and skin.

Eye signs

- *Multifocal, slate-gray episcleral pigmentation* (**Fig. 3.144**).
- *Ipsilateral iris hyperchromia* (**Fig. 3.145**).
- Choroidal hyperpigmentation in caucasians (**Fig. 3.146**).

- Melanoma of the uveal tract, orbit and optic nerve.
- Glaucoma.
- Iris mammillations.

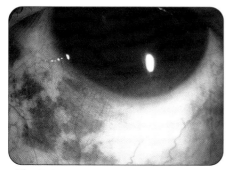

Fig. 3.144

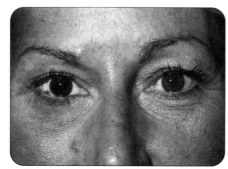

Fig. 3.145

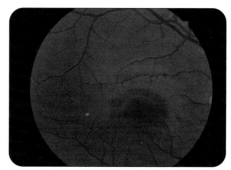

Fig. 3.146

OCULOCUTANEOUS ALBINISM

- This is an uncommon inborn error of metabolism which can be subdivided into two types according to whether or not the hair bulbs have tyrosinase activity.

- Inheritance is autosomal recessive.

Tyrosinase-negative

 ### Systemic features

- White hair and pink skin (**Fig. 3.147**).
- Absence of pigmented skin nevi.

 ### Associations

- Increased risk of skin squamous cell carcinoma.
- The chiasm has decreased number of uncrossed nerve fibers.
- Abnormal visual pathways from the lateral geniculate body to the occipital cortex.

 ### Eye signs

- Marked photophobia and severe impairement of visual acuity.
- Marked nystagmus which is usually pendular and horizontal.
- Gray to blue iris color with complete iris translucency (**Fig. 3.148**).
- Fundus hypopigmentation (**Fig. 3.149**).

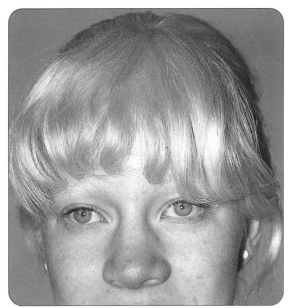

Fig. 3.147

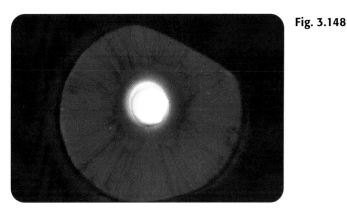

Fig. 3.148

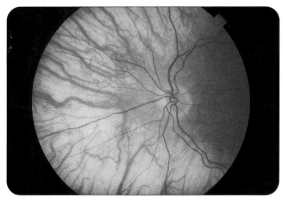

Fig. 3.149

Tyrosinase-positive

 Systemic features

- White or yellow tan hair color and white skin.
- Pigmented skin nevi may be present.

 Associations

- Increased risk of skin squamous cell carcinoma.

 Eye signs

- Variable photophobia and mild to moderate impairment of visual acuity.
- Mild to moderate nystagmus.
- Iris color is blue to yellow brown with variable degrees of iris translucency (**Fig. 3.150**).
- Variable fundus hypopigmentation.

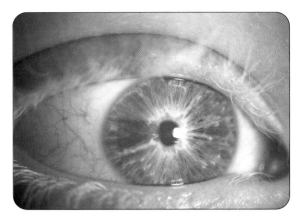

Fig. 3.150

OCULOPHARYNGEAL DYSTROPHY

- This is a rare myopathy.
- Inheritance is autosomal dominant.

- Ocular manifestations are universal.

Systemic features

 Presentation

- In adult life with dysphagia.

 Signs

- Weakness of pharyngeal muscles.
- Wasting of the temporalis muscle.

Eye signs

- Bilateral ptosis.

- Bilateral progressive external ophthalmoplegia.

ONCHOCERCIASIS

- This is caused by a filarial nematode, *Onchocerca volvulus*, which is transmitted by blackflies of the genus *Simulium*.

- Ocular manifestations are frequent and serious.

Systemic features

 Signs

- Dermatitis, mainly involving the midbody, characterized by pruritis and excoriation and later pigmentary changes and lichenification (**Fig. 3.151**).
- Subcutaneous nodules.
- Lymphadenopathy involving the femoral and inguinal nodes which may later result in elephantiasis.

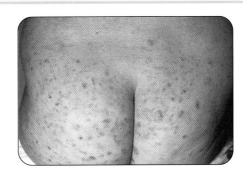

Fig. 3.151

Eye signs

- Punctate keratitis associated with microfilariae.
- Interstitial keratitis.
- Microfilariae in the anterior chamber.

- Anterior uveitis.
- Chorioretinitis with prominency of choroidal vessels.
- Optic neuritis.

OSTEOGENESIS IMPERFECTA

- This is a group of rare, inherited conditions of varying severity caused by defective fibrillary collagen type 1.

- Ocular manifestations are frequent but innocuous.

Type 1

Inheritance
- Autosomal dominant.

 Systemic features

- Few fractures with little or no deformity.
- Joint hyperextensibility.
- Normal stature.
- Aortic incompetence and mitral valve prolapse.

 Eye signs

- Blue sclera (**Fig. 3.152**).
- Corneal arcus.
- Megalocornea (**Fig. 3.153**).

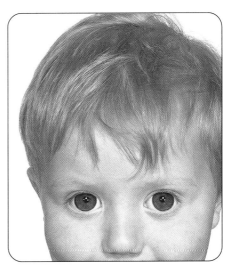

Fig. 3.153

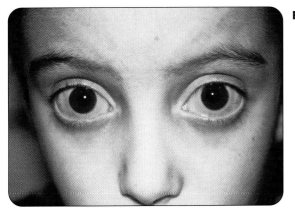

Fig. 3.152

Type 2

Inheritance
- Autosomal dominant.

 Systemic features

- Multiple fractures and short limbs (**Fig. 3.154**).
- Usually death in early infancy.

 Eye signs

- Blue sclera.

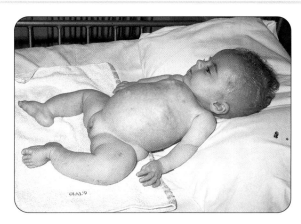

Fig. 3.154

Type 3

Inheritance
- Obscure.

 Systemic features

- Bones deform with age.
- Dental hypoplasia (dentinogenesis imperfecta).

- Triangular face with a large vault, prominent eyes and small jaw.

 Eye signs

- Blue sclera.

Type 4

Inheritance
- Autosomal dominant.

 Systemic features

- Moderate bony deformity and short stature.

Eye signs

- Normal sclera.

OXALOSIS

- This is rare inborn peroxismal disorder in which there is excessive oxalate production and systemic deposition caused by defective activity of alanine-glyoxylate amino-transferase.

- Inheritance is autosomal recessive.
- Ocular manifestations are frequent.

Systemic features

- Calcium oxalate deposition with secondary inflammation and damage.

- Involvement is principally of highly vascularized tissues such as the heart, bones and kidneys.

Eye signs

- *Crystalline retinopathy.*
- Later large geographic black lesions at the macula.

PAGET DISEASE

- This is an uncommon, idiopathic, metabolic bone disorder characterized by excessive and disorganized resorption and formation of bone.
- Ocular manifestations are infrequent.

Systemic features

 Presentation

- In adult life with a gradual onset of bone pain.

 Signs

- Enlargement, deformity and warmth of the skull (**Fig. 3.155**), pelvis and spine.

- Deformity of long bones with typical anterior bowing of the tibias (**Fig. 3.156**).

 Complications

- Arthropathy, kyphoscoliosis and fractures.
- Compression of the spine and cranial nerves.
- Deafness.
- Heart failure.
- Increased risk of osteosarcoma.

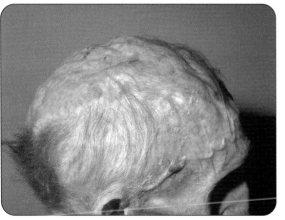

Fig. 3.155

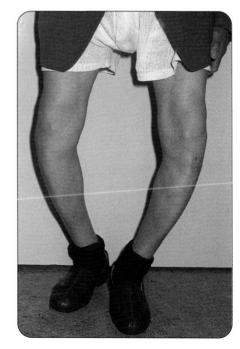

Fig. 3.156

Eye signs

- *Optic atrophy.*
- Proptosis.
- Ocular motor nerve palsies.
- Angioid streaks.

PANCREATITIS – ACUTE

- This is an uncommon condition which is associated with biliary disease and alcoholism.

- Ocular manifestations are infrequent.

Systemic features

 Presentation

- In adult life with a sudden onset of severe upper abdominal pain and vomiting.

 Signs

- Those are of the acute abdomen.

 Associations

- Liver disease.

Eye signs

- Retinal cotton-wool spots.

PEMPHIGOID

- This is an uncommon mucocutaneous blistering disease.

- Ocular manifestations are infrequent.

Systemic features

 Presentation

- In adult life.

 Signs

- Mucosal involvement is frequent.
- Large, symmetrical, widespread skin blisters (**Fig. 3.157**) which are usually self-limiting and resolve without scarring.

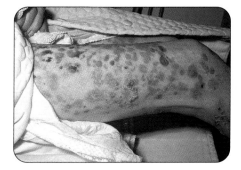

Fig. 3.157

Eye signs

- Cicatrizing conjunctivitis.

PEMPHIGUS VULGARIS

- This is an uncommon mucocutaneous blistering disease which equally affects the skin and mucosa.

- Ocular manifestations are infrequent.

Systemic features

 Presentation

- In adult life.

 Signs

- Initially involvement of the oral mucosa.
- Later widespread flaccid thin-walled cutaneous blisters (**Fig. 3.158**).

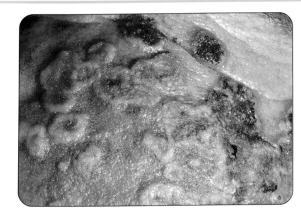

Fig. 3.158

Eye signs

- Conjunctivitis without scarring.

POLYARTERITIS NODOSA

- This is an uncommon, idiopthic, collagen vascular disease affecting medium-sized arteries in which aneurysm formation is a frequent occurrence.

- Ocular manifestations are infrequent but may be serious.

Eye signs

- *Keratoconjunctivitis sicca.*
- Corneal ulceration.

- Retinal vascular tortuosity.

ROSACEA

- This is a common skin disorder which affects the glabella, cheeks, nose and chin.

- Ocular manifestations are frequent.

Systemic features

 Presentation

- Usually in adult life with itching and flushing of facial skin.

 Signs

- Erythema progressing to telangiectasia (**Fig. 3.187**).
- Inflammatory papules and pustules (**Fig. 3.188**).
- Large inflammatory nodules, sebaceous gland hyperplasia (**Fig. 3.189**) and rhinophyma.

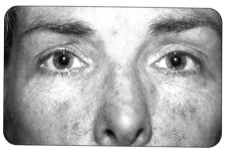

Fig. 3.187

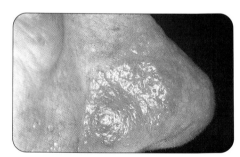

Fig. 3.188

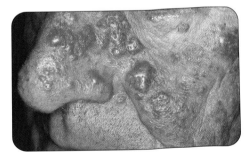

Fig. 3.189

Eye signs

- *Chronic posterior blepharitis* (**Fig. 3.190**).
- *Recurrent meibomian cysts* (**Fig. 3.191**).
- Conjunctivitis.
- Peripheral corneal thinning and vascularization (**Fig. 3.192**).

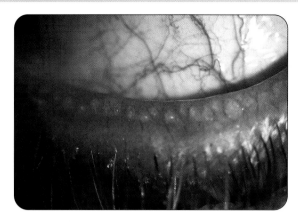

Fig. 3.190

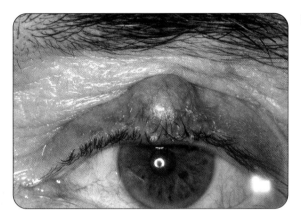

Fig. 3.191

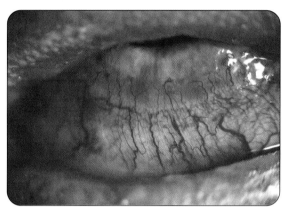

Fig. 3.192

SARCOIDOSIS

- This is a common, idiopathic multisystem granulomatous disease.

- Ocular manifestations are frequent and may be serious.

Systemic features

 Presentation

Acute-onset
This typically presents during the third decade in one of the following ways:
- Löfgren syndrome, which is characterized by fever, erythema nodosum, hilar lymphadenopathy and frequently arthralgia.

- Heerfordt syndrome (uveoparotid fever) which is characterized by fever, parotid gland enlargement and uveitis.
- Seventh nerve palsy which may be associated with other neurological features.

Insidious-onset
- This typically presents during the fifth decade with fatigue, dyspnea and arthralgia.

Signs

Lungs

There is pulmonary involvement in 90% of patients. The radiological staging is as follows:

- Stage 1 – bilateral hilar lymphadenopathy (**Fig. 3.193**).
- Stage 2 – bilateral hilar lymphadenopathy and reticulonodular parenchymal infiltrates (**Fig. 3.194**).
- Stage 3 – reticulonodular infiltrates alone (**Fig. 3.195**).
- Stage 4 – progressive pulmonary fibrosis with formation of bullae and bronchiectasis (**Fig. 3.196**).

Skin

- Erythema nodosum (**Fig. 3.197**).
- Granulomata.
- Lupus pernio (**Fig. 3.198**).

Neurological

- Cranial nerve palsies, most frequently facial (**Fig. 3.199**).
- Meningeal infiltration.
- Intracranial and intraspinal granulomas.

Other lesions

- Reticuloendothelial system.
- Liver.
- Kidneys.
- Bones.
- Heart.

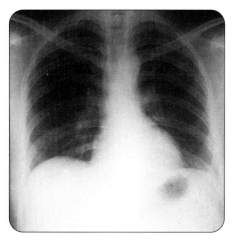

Fig. 3.193

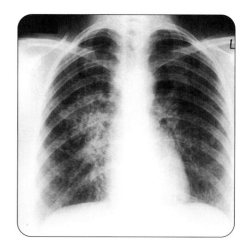

Fig. 3.194

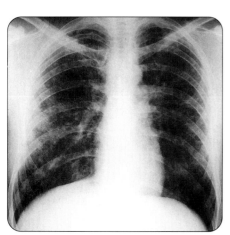

Fig. 3.195

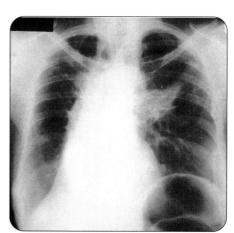

Fig. 3.196

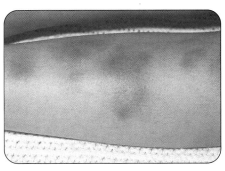

Fig. 3.197

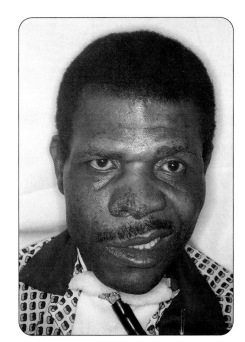

Fig. 3.199

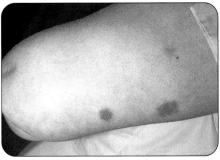

Fig. 3.198

Eye signs

Anterior segment
- Conjunctival granulomas (**Fig. 3.200**).
- Keratoconjunctivitis sicca.

Anterior uveitis
- Acute anterior uveitis typically affects patients with acute sarcoidosis.
- Chronic glanulomatous anterior uveitis (**Fig. 3.201**) typically affects older patients with chronic lung disease.

Vitreous
- Intermediate uveitis (**Fig. 3.202**).

Retina
- Periphlebitis which may be associated with 'candlewax drippings' (**Fig. 3.203**).
- Retinal and preretinal granulomas.
- Peripheral neovascularization.

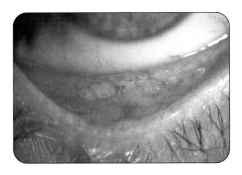

Fig. 3.200

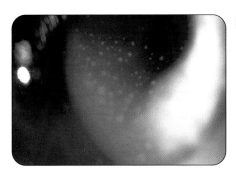

Fig. 3.201

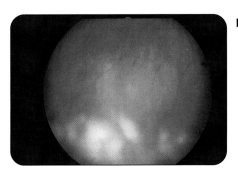

Fig. 3.202

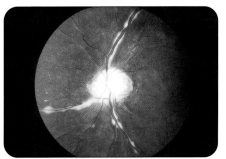

Fig. 3.203

Choroid
- Multifocal choroiditis (**Fig. 3.204**).
- Large, solitary granulomas which are rare.

Optic nerve head
- Focal granulomas (**Fig. 3.205**).
- Papilledema secondary to raised intracranial pressure.
- Disc neovascularization.

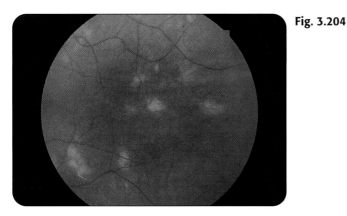

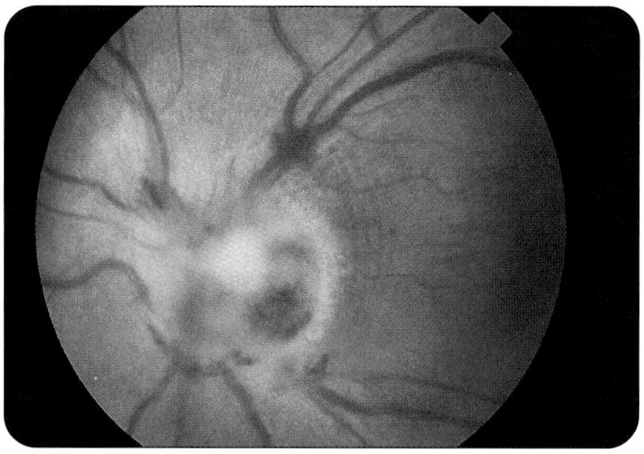

Fig. 3.204

Fig. 3.205

SCHILDER DISEASE

- This is a rare, relentlessly progressive demyelination indistinguishable from multiple sclerosis but with an earlier onset and a worse prognosis.
- Ocular manifestations are common.

Systemic features

- Onset is before age 10 years with death within 1 to 2 years.

Eye signs

- Bilateral optic neuritis without subsequent improvement.

SJÖGREN SYNDROME

- This is a common condition characterized by inflammation and destruction of lacrimal and salivary glands.
- The syndrome is classified as primary when it exists on its own, and secondary when it is associated with other disease such as rheumatoid arthritis, systemic lupus erythematosus, systemic sclerosis, polymyositis or primary biliary cirrhosis.
- It affects females much more frequently than males.
- Ocular manifestations are universal.

Systemic features

Presentation

- At any age from 15 to 65 with grittiness of the eyes and dryness of the mouth.

Signs

- Parotid enlargement with diminished saliva and a dry fissured tongue.
- Dry nasal passages.
- Diminished vaginal secretions and dyspareunia.

- Arthritis.
- Raynaud phenomenon.
- Cutaneous vasculitis.

Complications

- Reflux esophagitis and gastritis.
- Malabsorption due to pancreatic failure.
- Pulmonary disease.
- Multifocal neuropathy.
- Renal disease.

Eye signs

- *Keratoconjunctivitis sicca* (**Fig. 3.206**).
- Adie pupil.

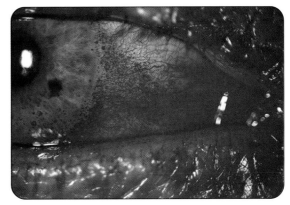
Fig. 3.206

STEVENS–JOHNSON SYNDROME (ERYTHEMA MULTIFORME MAJOR)

This is an uncommon, acute, serious but generally self-limiting mucocutaneous disease.
- The most common precipitating factors are a hypersensitivity reaction to drugs and infections caused by *Mycoplasma pneumoniae* and herpes implex virus.

- In over 50% of cases no cause can be found.
- Ocular manifestations are frequent.

Systemic features

 Presentation

- Usually between the third and fifth decades with fever, malaise, sore throat which last about 14 days.

 Signs

- Mucosal oral involvement characterized by bullae and erosions is universal and the lips show hemorrhagic crusting (**Fig. 3.207**).

- Mucosal genital involvement may also occur.
- Target skin lesions, consisting of a red centre which is itself encircles by a peripheral red ring, most frequently involve the palmar aspects of the hands and feet (**Fig. 3.208**).
- Skin blisters are usually transient but may be widespread and associated with hemorrhage and necrosis (**Fig. 3.209**).

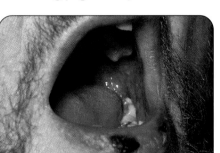
Fig. 3.207

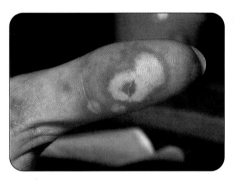
Fig. 3.208

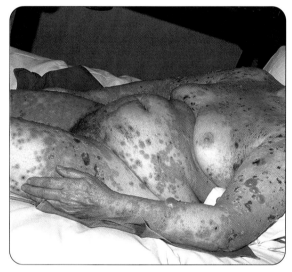
Fig. 3.209

Eye signs

- *Initially, transient membranous conjunctivitis* (**Fig. 3.210**).
- Later, conjunctival cicatrization may develop in some cases.

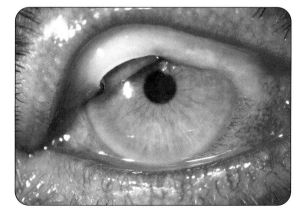
Fig. 3.210

STURGE–WEBER SYNDROME

- This is an uncommon, congenital condition which is one of the phacomatoses.

- Ocular manifestations are frequent.

Systemic features

Classification
- *Trisystem* form involving the face, leptomeninges and eyes.
- *Bisystem* form involving the face and eyes or the face and leptomeninges.

 Signs

- Facial nevus flammeus (port-wine stain) (**Fig. 3.211**).
- Ipsilateral parietal or occipital leptomeningeal hemangioma with contralateral hemiparesis and hemianopia.
- Epileptic fits.
- Mental retardation.

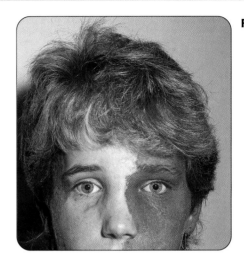

Fig. 3.211

Eye signs

- Glaucoma with optic disc cupping (**Fig. 3.212**) which is ipsilateral to the facial angioma.
- Ipsilateral episcleral hemangioma (**Fig. 3.213**).

- Ipsilateral diffuse choroidal hemangioma.
- Ipsilateral hemangioma of the iris and ciliary body.

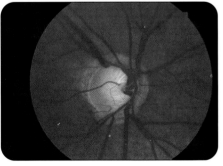

Fig. 3.212

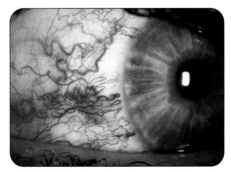

Fig. 3.213

SYPHILIS – ACQUIRED

- This is an infrequent sexually transmitted infection caused by the spirochete *Treponema pallidum*.

- Ocular manifestations are infrequent.

Systemic features

 Signs

Primary
- Painless ulcer (chancre).
- Regional lymphadenopathy.

Secondary
- Fever, malaise and generalized lymphadenopathy.
- Maculopapular rash involving the trunk (**Fig. 3.214**), or the palms and soles.
- Meningitis, nephritis and hepatitis.

Tertiary
- Aortitis.
- Tabes dorsalis and Charcot joints.
- Gummata in various organs.

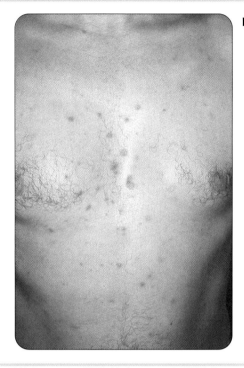

Fig. 3.214

Eye signs

Anterior
- Interstitial keratitis.
- Madarosis.
- Primary conjunctival chancre.
- Anterior uveitis.

Posterior
- Solitary or multifocal chorioretinitis.

- Retinal periarteritis which may result in optic atrophy and retinal scarring (**Fig. 3.215**).

Neuro-ophthalmic
- Neuroretinitis.
- Optic neuritis.
- Argyll Robertson pupils (**Fig. 3.216**).
- Ocular motor nerve palsies.

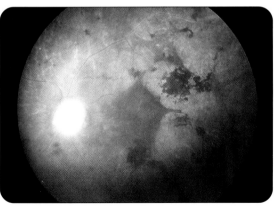

Fig. 3.215

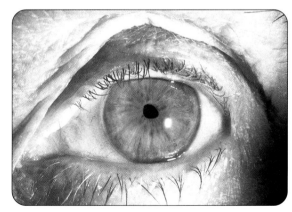

Fig. 3.216

SYPHILIS – CONGENITAL

- This uncommon infection with the spirochete *Treponema pallidum* is acquired *in utero*.

- Ocular manifestations are frequent but usually innocuous.

Systemic features

 Signs

Early
- Rhinitis and snuffles.
- Maculpapular rash especially on the buttocks and thighs.
- Fissures around the lips, nares and anus.
- Pneumonia.
- Hepatosplenomegaly and jaundice.
- Lymphadenopathy.

Late
- Sensorineural deafness.
- Frontal bossing.
- Saddle-shaped nasal deformity.
- Short maxilla and prognathous chin.
- High-arched palate.
- Malformed incisors (Hutchinson teeth) and mulberry molars.

Eye signs

- Anterior uveitis in early cases.
- Interstitial keratitis in late cases.
- Pigmentary retinopathy in late cases (**Fig. 3.217**).

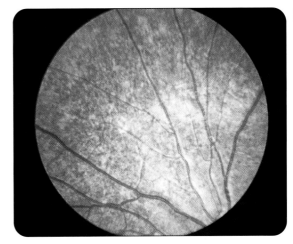

Fig. 3.217

SYRINGOMYELIA

- This is an uncommon neurological disease characterized by the presence of cavities surrounded by gliosis involving the crossing spinothalamic tracts in the region of the central canal of the spinal cord.

- Involvement of the medulla is termed syringobulbia.
- Ocular manifestations are infrequent.

Systemic features

 Presentation

- Usually in early adult life with an insidious onset of weakness and sensory loss initially involving the hands.

 Signs

- Sensory dissociation which is characterized by loss of pain and temperature but preservation of touch.
- Muscular wasting and weakness particularly of the small muscles of the hands.

- Syringobulbia may cause wasting of the tongue, dysphagia and vocal cord paralysis.

 Complications

- Scars from painless injuries.
- Charcot arthropathy.

Eye signs

- Horner syndrome.

SYSTEMIC LUPUS ERYTHEMATOSUS

- This is an uncommon, autoimmune, non-organ specific connective tissue disease characterized by widespread vasculitis.

- It affects females more commonly than males.
- Ocular manifestations are infrequent.

Systemic features

 Presentation

- Usually between in the third to fifth decades with undue fatiguability unassociated with any specific organ involvement.

 Signs

Mucocutaneous
- 'Butterfly' facial rash involving the cheeks and bridge of the nose (**Fig. 3.218**).
- Discoid rash.
- Vasculitis (**Fig. 3.219**).
- Telangiectasia.
- Alopecia and madarosis.
- Photosensitivity.
- Oral or nasopharyngeal ulceration.
- Raynaud phenomenon.

Musculoskeletal
- Arthritis which may resemble rheumatoid disease.
- Myositis.
- Tendonitis.

Renal
- Glomerulonephritis.

Cardiovascular
- Pericarditis, endocarditis and myocarditis.
- Arterial and venous occlusion.

Pulmonary
- Pleurisy.
- Pulmonary atelectasis and 'shrinking lungs'.

Hemopoietic
- Anemia.
- Thrombocytopenia, lymphopenia and leukopenia.
- Splenomegaly and lymphadenopathy.

Neurological
- Polyneuritis.
- Cranial nerve palsies.
- Spinal cord lesions.
- Epilepsy.
- Stroke.
- Psychosis.

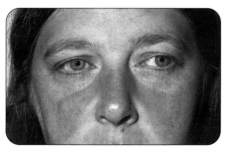
Fig. 3.218

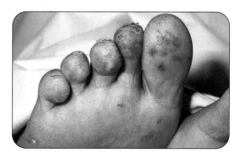
Fig. 3.219

Eye signs

- *Keratoconjunctivitis sicca.*
- *Peripheral ulcerative keratitis.*
- Madarosis.

- Retinal cotton-wool spots which may be associated with hemorrhages.
- Retinal periarteritis.
- Ischemic optic neuropathy.

SYSTEMIC MALIGNANCY – OCULAR SIGNS

Metastases

Orbital
- Proptosis (**Fig. 3.220**).
- Enophthalmos due to a scirrhous carcinoma.

Iris
- Iris mass which may be multiple.
- Irregular pupil.
- Spontaneous hyphema.

- Pseudo-hypopyon.
- Secondary glaucoma.

Choroid
- Placoid lesions at the posterior pole which may be multiple and bilateral (**Fig. 3.221**).

Central visual pathways
- Visual field defects.

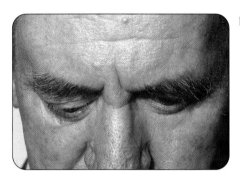

Fig. 3.220

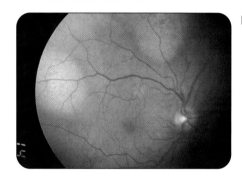

Fig. 3.221

Remote effects

Cancer-related retinopathy
This occurs in patients with epithelial tumors, most commonly small cell lung carcinoma. Occasionally it develops prior to the clinical diagnosis of the underlying carcinoma.

Signs
- Gradual onset of night-blindness (nyctalopia).
- Progressive visual loss and ring scotomas.
- Retinal degeneration with arteriolar attenuation and optic atrophy (**Fig. 3.222**).
- May lead to extinguished ERG.

Melanoma-related retinopathy
This occurs in patients with metastases from cutaneous melanomas (**Fig. 3.223**).

Signs
- Sudden onset of night blindness and shimmering photopsia.
- Constriction of visual fields.
- Flash ERG b-wave is reduced but a-wave amplitude is preserved.

Eaton–Lambert myasthenic syndrome
This most frequently occurs in association with small-cell bronchial carcinoma.

Signs
- Ptosis.
- Diplopia.

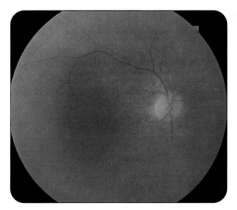

Fig. 3.222

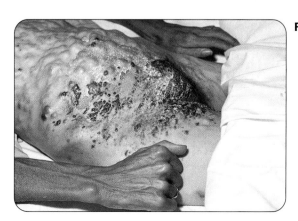

Fig. 3.223

Other causes of visual loss

- Meningeal infection by opportunistic organisms.

- Toxicity from radiation or chemotherapy.

SYSTEMIC SCLEROSIS

- This is a rare chronic connective tissue disease affecting the skin and internal organs which most frequently affects women.

- Ocular manifestations are infrequent and usually innocuous.

Systemic features

 Presentation

- Typically between the ages of 30 and 50 years with Raynaud phenomenon.

 Signs

- Skin tightening and thickening rise to a waxy appearance (**Fig. 3.224**).
- Subcutaneous fibrosis causing binding-down of facial skin and tapering of digits (sclerodactyly) (**Fig. 3.225**).
- Subcutaneous calcinosis (**Fig. 3.226**).
- Esophageal dysmobility.
- Involvement of the heart, lungs and kidneys.

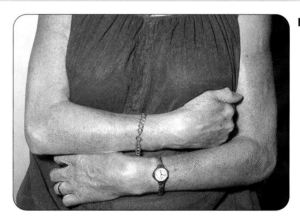

Fig. 3.224

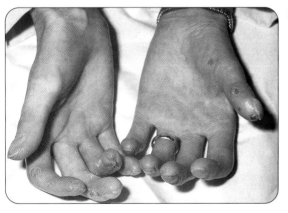

Fig. 3.225

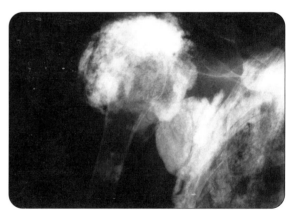

Fig. 3.226

Eye signs

- *Keratoconjunctivitis sicca.*

- Retinal cotton-wool spots and hemorrhages.

TANGIER DISEASE (ANALPHALIPOPROTEINEMIA)

- This is a rare metabolic disorder due to absence of high-density lipoprotein (HDL) resulting in the accumulation of cholesterol esters throughout the body.
- Inheritance is autosomal recessive.
- Ocular manifestations are frequent but innocuous.

Systemic features

 Signs

- Enlarged, orange–yellow tonsils and adenoids.

- Lymphadenopathy and hepatosplenomegaly.
- Thrombocytopenia.
- Neuropathy.

Eye signs

- Stromal corneal crystals.

TAKAYASU DISEASE

- This is a rare, idiopathic, granulomatous arteritis of the aorta and its main branches, as well as the pulmonary artery.
- It primarily affects Oriental women.
- Ocular manifestations are frequent.

Systemic features

 Presentation

- Usually in the third to fifth decades with an insidious onset of fatigue, fever, headache, syncope and dyspnea.

 Signs

- Asymmetric peripheral pulses or pulselessness.
- Wide differences in blood pressure between the arms.
- Arterial bruits.

Complications

- Infarction of the heart and bowel.
- Stroke.
- Renovascular hypertension.
- Aortic incompetence.
- Aortic aneurysm formation.
- Pulmonary hypertension.

Eye signs

- Slow-flow retinopathy.
- Ocular ischemic syndrome.

THYROTOXICOSIS (HYPERTHYROIDISM)

- This is a common autoimmune disease caused by excessive secretion of thyroid hormones by the entire thyroid gland.
- It affects women more commonly than men.
- Ocular manifestations are very frequent.

Systemic features

 Presentation

- Usually during the third and fourth decades with weight loss despite a good appetite, increased bowel frequency, sweating and heat intolerance, nervousness, irritability, palpitations, weakness and fatigue.

 Signs

External
- Thyroid enlargement (**Fig. 3.227**).
- Warm and sweaty skin with palmar erythema.

- Onycholysis affecting the finger nails, especially the ring fingers (Plummer's nails).
- Alopecia and vitiligo.
- Pretibial myxedema (**Fig. 3.228**).
- Clubbing of fingers (thyroid acropachy).
- Fine tremor and brisk tendon reflexes.
- Muscle weakness due to proximal myopathy.

Cardiovascular
- Sinus tachycardia, atrial fibrillation and premature ventricular beats.
- High output heart failure.

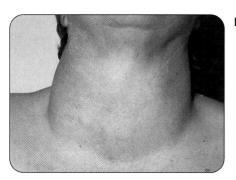

Fig. 3.227

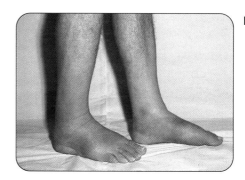

Fig. 3.228

Eye signs

Soft tissue
- Periorbital and lid swelling, and chemosis (**Fig. 3.229**).
- Superior limbic keratoconjunctivitis.
- Keratoconjunctivitis sicca.
- Dilated blood vessels over the horizontal rectus muscles.

Eyelid
- Retraction of upper eyelids in the primary gaze (Dalrymple sign) (**Fig. 3.230**).

- Retarded descent of upper eyelids in downgaze (lid lag – von Graefe sign) (**Fig. 3.231**).
- Retraction of the lower eyelids.

Proptosis
- May be unilateral, bilateral and asymmetrical (**Fig. 3.232**).
- May cause exposure keratopathy and corneal ulceration.
- May be associated with choroidal folds (**Fig. 3.233**).

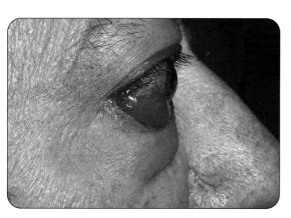

Fig. 3.229

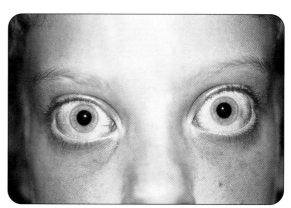

Fig. 3.230

Compressive optic neuropathy
- May occur in absence of significant proptosis.
- The disc may be normal, swollen or atrophic.

Restrictive myopathy
- Elevation defect is most common (**Fig. 3.234**).
- Abduction defect is second most common.
- Depression defect is next most common.
- Adduction defect is least common.

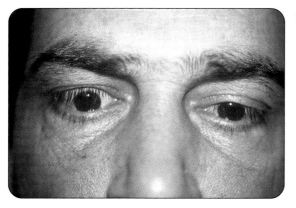

Fig. 3.231

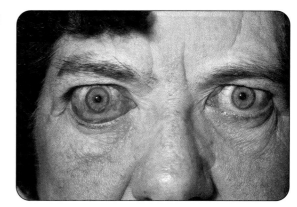

Fig. 3.232

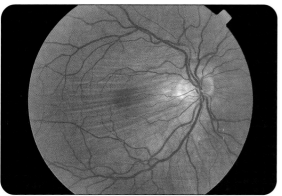

Fig. 3.233

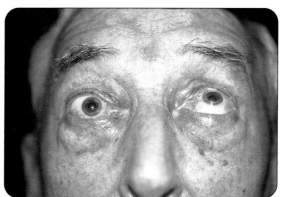

Fig. 3.234

TOXIC EPIDERMAL NECROLYSIS (LYELL DISEASE, SCALDED SKIN SYNDROME)

- This is a rare mucocutaneous disease characterized by acute epithelial necrosis which may be triggered by certain drugs or infections.

- Ocular manifestations are infrequent.

Systemic features

 Presentation

- In childhood or adult life with prodromal fever, cough, headache and malaise.

 Signs

- Mucosal blistering is universal.
- Transient, painful, widespread skin blisters resembling scalded skin (**Fig. 3.235**).
- Subsequent epidermal loss which can be precipitated by a lateral shearing force (Nikolsky sign).

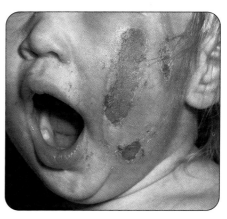

Fig. 3.235

Eye signs

- Mild cicatrizing conjunctivitis.

TOXOPLASMOSIS

- This is an infestation with an obligate intracellular protozoan, *Toxoplasma gondii*.

- Infestation is usually congenital (transplacental) and occasionally acquired.

Congenital

 Systemic features

- Stillbirth.
- Generalized convulsions, paralysis and hydrocephalus (**Fig. 3.236**).
- Intracranial calcification (**Fig. 3.237**).
- Visceral involvement.

 Eye signs

- Microphthalmos (**Fig. 3.238**).
- Bilateral macular scars in childhood (**Fig. 3.239**).
- Recurrent, unifocal retinitis adjacent to an old scar occurring later in life (**Fig. 3.240**).

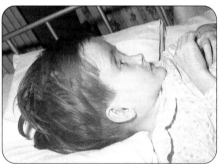

Fig. 3.236

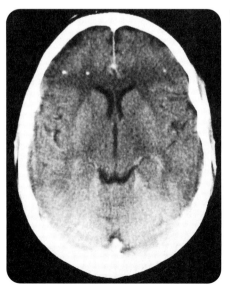

Fig. 3.237

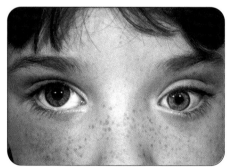

Fig. 3.238

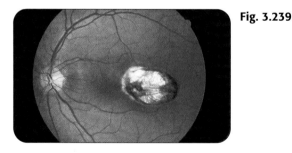

Fig. 3.239

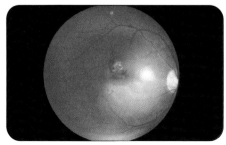

Fig. 3.240

Acquired

 Systemic features

In immunocompetent patients
- Frequently subclinical.
- Occasionally fever and lymphadenopathy.

In immunocompromised patients
- Intracerebral space-occupying lesion.

 Eye signs

- Retinitis which may be atypical and not adjacent to an old scar.

TUBERCULOSIS

- This is a common, chronic granulomatous infection caused by either bovine or human tubercule bacilli.
- Immunocompromised patients are at increased risk.

- Ocular manifestations are infrequent and only occur in post-primary infection.

Systemic features

 Presentation

- At any age with malaise, weight loss, night sweats, cough and hemoptysis.

 Signs

- Erythema nodosum.
- Fibrocaseous pulmonary disease.
- Lymph node involvement **(Fig. 3.241)**.
- Miliary hematogenous spread to many parts of the body.

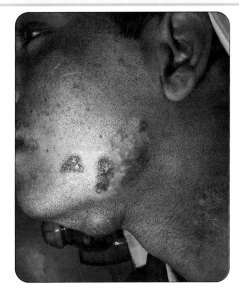

Fig. 3.241

Eye signs

- *Granulomatous anterior uveitis.*
- *Multifocal choroiditis.*

- Retinal periphlebitis.
- Solitary choroidal granuloma.

TUBEROUS SCLEROSIS (BOURNEVILLE DISEASE)

- The is a rare phacomatosis characterized by the triad of (a) epilepsy; (b) mental retardation; and (c) adenoma sebaceum.

- Inheritance is autosomal dominant but over 75% of cases are caused by a fresh mutation.
- Ocular manifestations are frequent but innocuous.

Systemic features

 Signs

Skin
- Adenoma sebaceum which are fibroangiomatous red papules that have a butterfly distribution around the nose and cheeks are universal (**Fig. 3.242**).
- Ash-leaf spots which are hypopigmented patches on the trunk, limbs and scalp. In infants with sparse skin pigmentation they are best detected using ultraviolet light (Wood's lamp).
- Shagreen patches which consist of diffuse thickening over the lumbar region.

- Fibrous plaques on the forehead.
- Skin tags (molluscum fibrosum pendulum).

CNS
- Astrocytic cerebral hamartomas are universal (**Fig. 3.243**).
- Cortical tubers.

Visceral hamartomas
- Renal angiomyolipomas.
- Cardiac rhabdomyomas.
- Subungual hamartomas (**Fig. 3.244**).

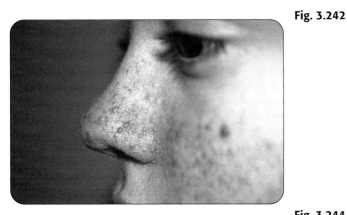

Fig. 3.242

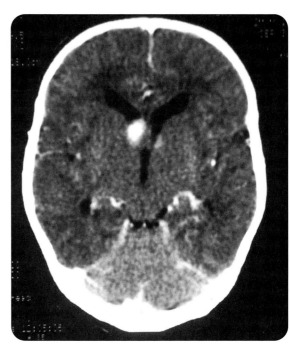

Fig. 3.243

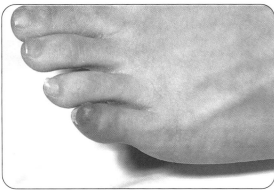

Fig. 3.244

Eye signs

- Retinal astrocytomas in 50% of patients which are bilateral in about 15% (**Fig. 3.245**).

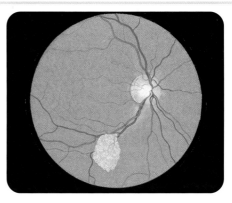

Fig. 3.245

TUBULOINTERSTITIAL NEPHRITIS

- This is an uncommon hypersensitivity reaction to a drug.

- Ocular manifestations are frequent.

Systemic features

 Presentation

- Fatigue, anorexia and weight loss.

 Signs

- Anemia.
- Hypertension.
- Non-oliguric renal failure.

Eye signs

- Bilateral non-granulomatous anterior uveitis.

TURCOT SYNDROME

- This is a rare condition which is associated with familial adenomatous polyposis.

- Inheritance is autosomal dominant.
- Ocular manifestations are frequent.

Systemic features

 Signs

- Asymptomatic adenomatous polyposis in which the colon, rectum and duodenum are affected by hundreds or often thousands of polyps.
- Tumors involving the central nervous system, particularly medulloblastoma and glioblastoma.

Associations

- Increased risk of carcinoma of the colon and less frequently of the duodenum.

Eye signs

- Multiple, frequently bilateral, areas of atypical congenital hypertrophy of the retinal pigment epithelium.

TURNER SYNDROME

- This is an uncommon, chromosomal disorder (XO with 45 chromosomes) which is characterized by gonadal dysgenesis.

- Ocular manifestations are infrequent.

Systemic features

 Signs

- Short hirsute female.
- Sexual infantilism.
- Webbed and short neck (**Fig. 3.246**).
- Cubitus valgus.
- Broad chest with widely spaced nipples.
- Multiple pigmented nevi.
- Renal anomalies.

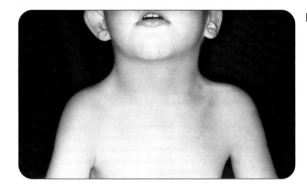

Fig. 3.246

Eye signs

- Keratoconus.

- Blue sclera.

ULCERATIVE COLITIS

- This is an uncommon, idiopathic, chronic, relapsing inflammatory disease, involving the rectum and extending proximally to involve part or all of the large intestine (**Fig. 3.247**).
- Patients with longstanding disease carry an increased risk of developing carcinoma of the colon.
- Ocular manifestations are infrequent.

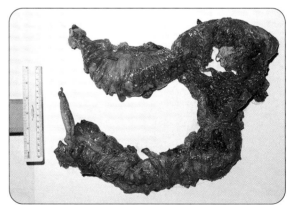

Fig. 3.247

Systemic features

 Presentation

- Usually in adult life with a diarrhea with blood and mucus, lower abdominal cramps, urgency and tenesmus.
- Constitutional symptoms include tiredness, weight loss, malaise and fever.

 Signs

- Aphthous mouth ulceration.
- Erythema nodosum.
- Pyoderma gangrenosum (**Fig. 3.248**).
- Finger clubbing.

 Associations

- Asymmetrical lower limb arthritis.
- Sacroiliitis and ankylosing spondylitis.

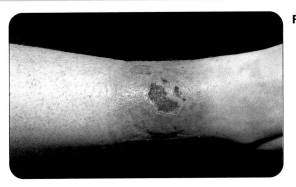

Fig. 3.248

 Complications

- Autoimmune hepatitis.
- Sclerosing cholangitis.
- Arterial and venous thrombosis.
- Carcinoma of the colon.

Eye signs

- *Acute anterior uveitis.*
- Peripheral corneal infiltrates.

- Conjunctivitis.

USHER SYNDROME

- This term encompasses a group of rare, genetic disorders characterized by visual loss and deafness.

- Inheritance is autosomal recessive.

Usher 1 (three subtypes)

 Systemic features

- Congenital, severe hearing loss with absent vestibular function.

 Eye signs

- Pigmentary retinopathy (**Fig. 3.249**).

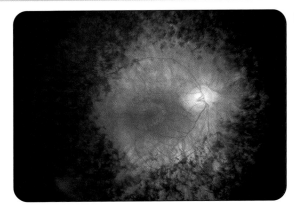

Fig. 3.249

Usher 2 (two subtypes)

 Systemic features

- Congenital, moderate-severe hearing loss with normal vestibular function.

 Eye signs

- Pigmentary retinopathy.

Usher 3

 Systemic features

- Progressive hearing loss.

Eye signs

- Pigmentary retinopathy.

VOGT–KOYANAGI–HARADA SYNDROME

- This is an idiopathic, multisystem disorder which typically affects pigmented individuals and the Japanese.

- Ocular manifestations are universal.
- The syndrome can be subdivided as follows:

Vogt–Koyanagi syndrome

 Systemic features

- Alopecia, poliosis and vitiligo (**Fig. 3.250**).

 Eye signs

- Chronic granulomatous anterior uveitis.

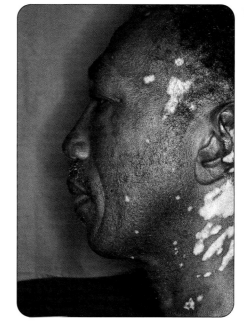

Fig. 3.250

Index